Understanding Hepatitis,

James L. Achord, M.D.

University Press of Mississippi
Jackson

www.upress.state.ms.us

Copyright © 2002 by University Press of Mississippi
All rights reserved
Manufactured in the United States of America
Illustrations by Regan Causey Tuder
10   09   08   07   06   05   04   03   02   4   3   2   1
∞

Library of Congress Cataloging-in-Publication Data

Achord, James L.
    Understanding hepatitis / James L. Achord.
        p. cm.—(Understanding health and sickness series).
    Includes bibliographical references and index.
    ISBN 1-57806-435-X (cloth : alk. paper)—ISBN 1-57806-436-8
(paper : alk. paper)
    1. Hepatitis—Popular works. I. Title. II. Series.
RC848.H42 A26 2002
616.3'623—dc21   2001049243

British Library Cataloging-in-Publication Data available

Contents

Introduction

"Infectious hepatitis" has plagued humanity for millennia. The disease that we now call hepatitis A was recognized in antiquity; references to it can be found in the writings of Hippocrates (ca. 400 B.C.E.), in the Talmud, and in ancient Chinese medical texts. Outbreaks of jaundice were seen in the seventeenth, eighteenth, and nineteenth centuries, especially in military campaigns where crowded and unsanitary conditions were common. In fact, the condition became known as "campaign disease." Epidemics of infectious hepatitis hit hard during Napoleon's Egyptian campaign, the Civil War, and the British drive in Mesopotamia in World War I. During World War II, more than 150,000 U.S. soldiers and over 5 million German army and civilian personnel were incapacitated by hepatitis. Outbreaks during the Korean and Vietnam conflicts felled thousands of U.S. troops. Epidemics in civilian populations on all continents have been and continue to be common.

The word "hepatitis" is made up of the prefix "hepat-," from the Greek, referring to anything pertaining to the liver, and the suffix "-itis," which means inflammation. Therefore, "hepatitis" means inflammation of the liver. There are many causes, including several viruses, a host of chemicals and drugs, bacteria, diseases of the immune system, inherited factors, and herbs. When people (including physicians) say "hepatitis," they are usually referring to the sort caused by viruses. That will be our major concern in this book, although many of the nonviral types will also be mentioned.

Viral hepatitis is common in developed nations such as the United States but even more so in other parts of the world. Men and women are equally susceptible to infection. The disease is seen more often in lower socioeconomic groups. Seven known viruses—named A, B, C, D, E, G, and TTV (transfusion transmitted virus)—primarily infect the liver, but only the first four are of any concern in the United States. Hepatitis caused by these four will be discussed in some detail.

Every year, about 140,000 people in the United States have acute hepatitis A, and there are perhaps over 1,000,000 cases around the world. Fortunately, hepatitis A does not cause chronic hepatitis, defined as disease that lasts longer than six months. In the United States there are about 1,250,000 people infected with hepatitis B, many of whom have chronic disease, while worldwide about 350,000,000 are infected. Hepatitis C is unique in many ways and is virtually always chronic. Today some 4,000,000 people in the United States, or 1.6 percent of the population, have been infected with this virus at some time in the past, and at least three out of four of those have live virus in their blood. The infection rate has decreased dramatically in recent years. In 1988 the Centers for Disease Control and Prevention estimated that there were 230,000 new cases of hepatitis C, but by 1996 the number was down to 36,000. The worldwide prevalence of chronic hepatitis C is around 150,000,000 to 170,000,000 people (probably an underestimation). The fourth virus, hepatitis D, is uncommon in the United States.

Viruses G and TTV are common, but, although the liver is probably the primary site of infection, studies indicate little or no damage, and they are not believed to be of concern.

More often than not there are no signs or symptoms of acute infection. In those who do become ill, hepatitis may make itself known by jaundice, a yellow discoloration of tissues and best seen in the whites of the eyes and in the skin. A common term for hepatitis is the redundant phrase "yellow jaundice." At first the disease was thought to be caused by plugging of the bile ducts by mucus, but in 1839 it was recognized to be the result of disease of liver cells. Not until about a hundred years later (only sixty years ago) was the infectious agent recognized as a virus. That there was more than one kind of liver virus was learned from experiments with volunteers during and after World War II and in remarkable studies of institutionalized children in the 1950s and 1960s, but it has only been in the past thirty years or so that studies have identified and characterized the specific viruses that primarily attack the liver.

Because viral hepatitis sometimes has serious acute and chronic consequences, reference to it tends to raise great and usually unreasonable fears of death or disability, whereas in fact the majority who become infected do quite well without any complications or long-term effects. Newspapers, of course, report the unfortunate ones, usually celebrities, who have poor outcomes and sometimes require liver transplantation. The risk of serious complications varies greatly with the type of hepatitis.

The purpose of this book is to discuss the various forms of hepatitis in comprehensible terms so as provide the reader with a better understanding of the disease. The focus is on the more common viral diseases, but some of the nonviral causes are also covered. Current research efforts are described in the final chapter.

Understanding Hepatitis

I. The Liver and Hepatitis

The liver has been variously described as the seat of the soul, the source of emotions, and a predictor of the future. It is the body's largest single organ and is necessary for life (fig 1.1). This vital organ is a domed solid structure with a relatively flat bottom surface to which the gallbladder is attached. It nestles against the diaphragm in the right upper portion of the abdominal cavity. It is protected by the right lower ribs but can usually be felt in the abdomen just beneath the ribs when a deep breath is taken and the diaphragm flattens, pushing down on the liver. It has two major lobes,

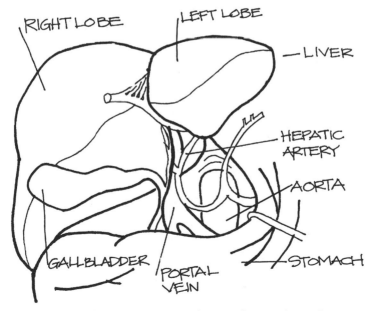

FIG. 1.1. The under side of the liver showing the portal vein (beneath the stomach) and position of the gallbladder.

a large right one and a much smaller left one. It weighs between 1.2 and 1.8 kilograms (about 2 1/2 to 4 pounds), with
a woman's weighing about 0.5 kilograms (a pound or so)
less than a man's. The liver receives a tremendous amount of
blood (about two-thirds of the amount propelled by each beat
of the heart) from two sources, the main one being the portal
vein, with a much smaller amount coming through the hepatic
artery. The hepatic artery carries highly oxygenated blood
and provides that essential element to the liver. The portal
vein collects all blood that comes from the gut and pancreas
(fig. 1.2). Thus, the liver receives all substances absorbed from
the gut. One can say that the liver "sits in the middle of the
bloodstream," because all blood circulates through it several
times each hour. The portal vein divides into smaller and
smaller vessels within the liver (fig. 1.3). The smallest ones,
called sinusoids, are somewhat larger than capillaries, and
carry blood that bathes liver cells. After going through the

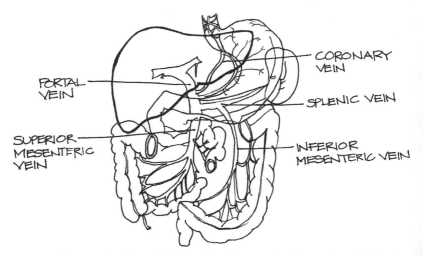

FIG. 1.2. The portal vein and its branches. The portal vein receives all blood
from the gut via the superior and inferior mesenteric veins. The splenic vein
joins the portal vein near the liver, shown in outline.

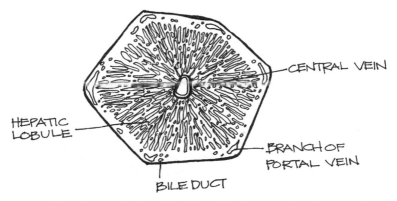

CENTRAL VEIN

HEPATIC LOBULE

BRANCH OF PORTAL VEIN

BILE DUCT

FIG. 1.3 The microcirculation of the liver. Blood enters from the portal vein, percolates through the sinusoids, where it is exposed to liver cells, and empties into the central vein (central to liver lobule), which is also called the peripheral vein because it is farther away from the heart in terms of blood flow.

sinusoids, blood is collected into six central veins and then into larger and larger veins until it reaches the major outflow vessel of the liver, the hepatic vein. This vein empties directly into the right side of the heart, where blood is pumped through the lungs, from there into the left side of the heart, and then throughout the body.

Liver cells are arranged in a six-sided pattern that resembles a berry. These groups of liver cells are arranged in larger groups called lobules, or small lobes. Each lobule is supplied by blood from the portal vein and hepatic artery. The tract these vessels traverse within the liver is called the portal area. It is while blood is circulating through the sinusoids that there is mutual exchange of substances between the liver cells and blood.

Bile is made by liver cells. It contains waste products removed from blood, such as bilirubin, and excretes them into tiny bile ducts (see fig. 1.3). These small ducts empty into larger and larger ducts from each lobe of the liver and finally

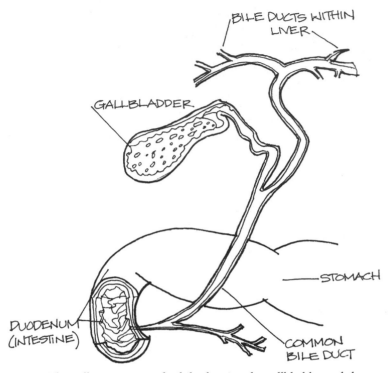

Fig. 1.4. The collection system for bile showing the gallbladder and the entrance of the common bile duct into the gut just beyond the stomach.

join as the common bile duct (fig. 1.4). The common bile duct empties into the first portion of the gut.

The liver has a remarkable capacity to regenerate itself. Damaged cells are rapidly replaced. Surgical removal of as much as two-thirds of the liver will result in regeneration of a mass of liver within weeks that is equal to the original mass.

Liver Functions

The liver performs a large number of functions that are essential to life. It is central to energy homeostasis through its metabolism of nutrients and manufactures substances that cause blood to clot (coagulate) as well as those that prevent inappropriate clotting. It removes certain waste products, metabolizes a host of drugs, traps and kills any bacteria that are in the blood, and removes toxic secretions of bacteria, as well as absorbed but unusable substances.

The liver processes a large number of amino acids (which make up proteins), both those absorbed from the gut and those made in the body by tissues other than the liver. For the purposes of this discussion, it will be useful to explain the role of the liver in the production of several substances.

Albumin is an important protein made only in the liver. It serves as a good example of all protein production. DNA in the nucleus copies a portion of itself containing instructions (via the pattern of amino acids making up this portion) onto a strand of messenger RNA (mRNA). The mRNA leaves the nucleus and moves into the cytoplasm of the cell. When it encounters the "manufacturing plant" of the cell, called a ribosome, mRNA attaches to it and the ribosome begins to make whatever protein is called for—in this case, albumin. This protein is a carrier or transporter for smaller proteins, some chemicals (including many drugs), and some waste products. It circulates in blood where it makes up about half of all the protein present. Its half-life is about twenty days; that is, half the albumin present at any time has been used up in twenty days and replaced with newly made albumin. It is a component of fluid in tissue. Since it is made only in the liver and has a relatively short half-life, interference with its manufacture results in a precipitous fall in its concentration in serum. Its production is an exception to the large reserve capacity of the liver. In general terms, the liver can increase its albumin production by not more than twofold. Measurement of the level of albumin in serum is therefore an important indicator of liver function.

Circulating albumin releases its load to the appropriate cells, including hepatic cells, for processing. It causes water to move into and remain in blood by osmosis, thus preventing circulating blood from becoming too concentrated. If albumin concentration in blood is very low, water tends to move from blood into tissue. This fluid can be seen as swelling (edema), especially of the feet and legs, or as an accumulation in the abdominal cavity (ascites). The normal level of serum albumin is 3.3 to 4.5 milligrams per milliliter (mg/mL). Edema or ascites usually does not occur until the level in serum is less than 2.5 mg/mL.

Ammonia is an important nitrogen-containing compound that is a product of protein metabolism. Its nitrogen is used by many tissues in the production of other proteins. The liver is the major site of ammonia metabolism; it is converted there into urea and either eliminated by the kidneys through urine or used for the production of more complex proteins. If liver function is severely compromised, ammonia is taken up by the liver and metabolized more slowly than normal. It thus accumulates in serum, where it interferes with normal brain function (see hepatic encephalopathy in chapter 2). Although not practical for clinical use, measurements of the rate of uptake of ammonia and of urea production can be used to measure liver function.

Bacteria normally living in the colon are an important source of ammonia, which is a by-product of their metabolism. The ammonia they produce is absorbed directly across the colon wall into the portal vein and thence to the liver. Interference with bacterial metabolism significantly reduces blood ammonia levels.

The liver is the major source of prothrombin, a protein precursor to thrombin, which is essential for blood clotting. The amount of prothrombin in blood is measured by determining how fast blood clots in a test tube when all other essential factors are added. This is called the prothrombin time. Normal prothrombin time is twelve seconds. A deficiency of prothrombin results in a prolonged prothrombin time. If the level of prothrombin becomes extremely low, minor trauma is followed by unexpected bleeding and even spontaneous bleeding into the skin (bruising). At least thirteen proteins produced by the liver are essential for the complex process of blood clotting, also referred to as coagulation. At least five proteins produced by the liver prevent inappropriate clotting within blood vessels. Prothrombin is the easiest to measure, and the others will not be discussed. Essential to the production of prothrombin is vitamin K, a deficiency of which also causes a prolonged prothrombin time. Any spontaneous reduction in prothrombin level in blood usually reflects abnormal liver function. Fortunately, the liver can make much more prothrombin than needed if called upon to do so. In fact, well over two-thirds of the liver can be too sick to function before the level of prothrombin in blood is reduced, the remaining normal cells making up the deficit. A markedly low level of prothrombin in acute hepatitis, regardless of the cause, is a serious prognostic sign because it reflects extensive and often irreversible liver injury. If the amount of prothrombin is sufficiently reduced, clotting is slowed or fails to occur.

In any tissue injury, prothrombin is converted to thrombin, causing blood to clot, thus sealing the area and preventing blood loss. If clotting occurs in a larger vessel, blood flow stops until the clot is dissolved by natural defense mechanisms. In acute thrombophlebitis or an acute heart attack (myocardial infarction), clotting of blood within blood vessels has occurred. In such instances, it is desirable to inhibit clotting in order to prevent formation of additional clots. This is routinely done with drugs such as warfarin, a common form of which is Coumadin. Warfarin (also the active ingredient in some rat poisons) is a direct antagonist to vitamin K. Therefore, carefully controlled doses of warfarin effectively prevent vitamin K from serving its essential role in the production of prothrombin, the level of which falls.

Oxygen is transported to tissue by hemoglobin, the red in red blood cells. These cells have a life span of about 120 days.

As they die, more red cells are produced in bone marrow; if there are too few red cells, a person is said to be anemic. The breakdown product of hemoglobin is a waste product called bilirubin, a yellow pigment. Bilirubin is taken up by the liver, processed, and secreted into bile. Uptake, processing, and secretion of bilirubin are energy-requiring functions. If for any reason liver cells cannot process bilirubin (as in hepatitis) or there is blockage of the bile ducts, this yellow pigment accumulates in blood and is deposited in most body tissues. When bilirubin is visible, jaundice is present. Jaundice also occurs when there is disease (e.g., hemolytic anemia) in which red cells break down so rapidly that even the normal liver cannot process the released bilirubin fast enough. Normal serum bilirubin is less than 1.2 mg/mL. Jaundice is best seen in the whites of the eyes but not before the serum bilirubin is above 3 mg/mL.

The liver is central to energy homeostasis of the body. Energy is taken into the body in the form of food, made up of carbohydrates, proteins, and fat. Virtually all of these must be processed into less complex compounds that can be moved across cell membranes and used for energy. The liver not only breaks down absorbed carbohydrates into simple sugars, including glucose, a major source of energy used by most cells of the body, but manufactures glucose from a number of simple proteins and lipids (fat), a process known as gluconeogenesis. The liver stores glucose not immediately needed by converting it into a complex carbohydrate called glycogen. Glycogen can be readily converted into glucose within the liver. Muscle cells can also store glycogen and, unlike most other tissues, use it directly for energy. Between meals, glucose in blood continues to be used for energy, and blood levels tend to fall. Blood sugar levels are maintained by conversion of glycogen back to glucose, a process called glycogenolysis. This process makes available a constant supply of energy for the whole body. A sign of extensive liver damage is the inability of the liver to maintain blood glucose levels by glycogenolysis, resulting in low blood sugar levels. Since the brain uses only glucose for its energy source, very low blood glucose levels result in unconsciousness and convulsions. To prevent low blood sugar levels in severe hepatitis, it may be necessary to continuously infuse glucose intravenously.

Cholesterol, in addition to being absorbed from the diet, is also made in the liver. It is vital to living tissue because it is an essential component of cell membranes, and from it are made a number of essential vitamins, hormones, and bile salts. Excess cholesterol is excreted by the liver into bile and then eliminated in stool. (A discussion of the complex reactions necessary for the balance of cholesterol in the body is beyond the scope of this book.) In disease of liver cells, serum cholesterol tends to fall because its manufacture is inhibited, whereas in obstruction to bile flow in bile ducts the level tends to increase, since it cannot be eliminated. Examination of these changes in serum cholesterol levels is sometimes helpful to a physician who is making decisions about the cause of jaundice.

Bile produced by the liver also contains bile salts, which are made within liver cells and secreted into bile; they are essential in the breakdown and digestion of dietary fats. Bile is collected within the liver into tiny tubes that empty into larger bile ducts, finally becoming one common bile duct that collects all bile (see fig. 1.2) and empties into the upper gut. The gallbladder branches off the common duct and stores bile until it is released during meals. The gallbladder is attached to the under surface of the liver and lies close to the muscles of the front of the abdomen.

Gallstones are formed when bile salts and cholesterol are so concentrated that they cannot remain dissolved in gallbladder fluid and precipitate out as crystals. Crystals then join together to form stones. If these stones pass out of the gallbladder and become lodged in the common duct, bile cannot reach the intestinal tract, and the individual becomes jaundiced. This type of obstructive jaundice is, of course, not related to the jaundice caused by disease of hepatic cells such as in hepatitis.

Enzymes are complex proteins produced by every living cell. There are thousands of these substances which catalyze chemical reactions in the body, and each enzyme catalyzes specific reactions. Small amounts of enzymes normally cross the membrane that surrounds each liver cell and enter the blood where they can be measured. The levels of enzyme in serum represent the sum of the events surrounding millions of cells. It is not necessary to know the specific function of these enzymes to understand how changes in blood levels help physicians to discover liver disease and discern its type. If liver cell membranes are injured, as with inflammation, more of these enzymes "leak" into the blood, and their levels are higher than normal. When damaged cells recover or are replaced by normal cells, the blood levels of these enzymes return to normal. While the liver produces thousands of enzymes, three are especially important indicators of diseases of the liver—alanine transaminase, aspartate transaminase, and alkaline phosphatase.

Alanine Transaminase (ALT) and Aspartate Transaminase (AST)

The serum aminotransferases were previously called trans-aminases. Alanine aminotransferase (ALT) was called serum glutamic-pyruvic transaminase, or SGPT, and aspartate amino-transferase (AST) was called serum glutamic-oxaloacetic transaminase, or SGOT. Only the names have changed. SGPT is still sometimes used instead of ALT and SGOT instead of the preferred AST. Physicians considering liver disease as the cause of a health problem measure blood levels of these three enzymes in liver function tests. While found in smaller amounts in other organs, ALT is present in large amounts in the liver. Therefore, when a larger-than-normal amount is present in the blood, it is probably coming from damaged liver cells. While AST is also made in large amounts in the liver, it is also made in several other organs, such as muscles. Thus, elevated levels of AST in the blood could be coming from the liver or from other organs. This is why more attention is paid to the levels of ALT than of AST in known or suspected liver disease although both are usually measured simultaneously.

Blood levels of ALT and AST reported vary with the machines used to measure them. Results are always given with the established normal limits for that particular machine. The usual upper limits of normal for ALT are either about forty or seventy international units/mL and somewhat less for AST. Once liver disease is known to be present, elevated blood levels are looked upon as evidence of active hepatic cell injury. The degree of elevation does not necessarily indicate the degree of total cell damage, and the level of blood enzyme does not reliably indicate the likelihood of recovery. For example, a blood ALT level of three thousand does not mean that recovery is less likely than if the level is three hundred (compared to a normal level of seventy). In fact, a rapid fall in ALT from abnormal to normal levels can mean either that the liver cells are recovering, as is usually the case, or that the cells have completely ceased functioning and are no longer able to make the enzyme.

Alkaline Phosphatase

This enzyme is also made in many tissues of the body, but the two sources that contribute to what is found in the blood are bones and the liver. Blood levels become elevated if there is obstruction to the flow of bile or if there is bone destruction and repair. Therefore, if the blood level is elevated, the physician must distinguish between these two sources. For this purpose, two serum enzymes, gamma glutamyl transaminase (GGT) and 5'nucleotidase, are useful since they are produced in the liver but not in bone. GGT is more commonly measured by clinicians than is 5'nucleotidase. If both the GGT (or 5'nucleotidase) and the alkaline phosphatase levels are elevated, the source must be the liver. Conversely, if the alkaline phosphatase is elevated but the GGT or 5'nucleotidase is normal, the source of the alkaline phosphatase is not the liver. The production of these enzymes by the liver increases when there is any obstruction to the flow of bile, and increased amounts appear in the blood. While elevation of the serum alkaline phosphatase level nearly always occurs with obstruction, such as that due to stones or tumors, it may also occur to a much lesser degree when hepatic cells become infected and swollen, closing off small bile ducts.

Causes of Hepatitis

Although most people who speak of hepatitis mean inflammation of the liver caused by viruses, there are many other causes. Perhaps a word about the nature of viruses would be helpful. In contrast to bacteria, which can be seen under the microscope, viruses are submicroscopic. To reproduce, they must reside in living cells, although they can survive (but not reproduce) outside of living cells. While antibiotics have no effect on viruses, there are some drugs that inhibit them, and others are in development. Viruses "highjack" the metabolic processes of the cells in which they grow, causing the host cells to manufacture the proteins necessary for virus reproduction. The immune system produces antibodies against the virus, but this takes time, and, in the interim, the virus is reproducing rapidly. Most viruses do not destroy the cell in which they reside, but they do cause injury leading to inflammation.

Inflammation may be obvious, with fever, pus, and abscess formation, or may be subtle with little or no fever or other symptoms. The latter is more likely in diseases caused by viruses. The inflammatory process tends to rid the body of the causes as well as the products of cell injury, including the debris of killed body cells. In this response to injury, normal cells may also be destroyed.

Inflammation is a complex process that is initiated by tissue injury, whatever the cause. Tissue injury of any sort initiates the inflammatory reaction with which we are all familiar. In vigorous bacterial inflammation, local release of nitrous oxide causes dilation of blood vessels, with subsequent increase in blood flow, and the area becomes warm. Further, the linings of blood vessels are damaged, and blood coagulation within vessels tends to isolate the area, preventing spread of infection. In the less vigorous inflammatory reaction initiated by many virus infections, including those causing hepatitis, the signs and symptoms of inflammation may be mild and go unrecognized.

Multiple substances are released at the site of injury. Specific lymphocytes, called T cells (as well as specialized T cells called killer T cells), and B cells are attracted. T lymphocytes and B lymphocytes are named for their origins, the thymus and bone marrow, respectively. After infancy, T cells are made in the bone marrow also. The primary function of T cells is to recognize proteins that are not part of the host ("self" proteins) and to engulf and destroy them; this is called cellular immunity. T cells also may directly attack host cells, the membranes of which have been altered by viruses, bacteria, trauma, or some other agent and are therefore not recognized as "self" antigens. The function of B lymphocytes is to manufacture antibodies against foreign protein or antigens; this is called humoral immunity and was the first type of immunity to be identified. Antibodies that develop after an initial infection are IgM antibodies, while those that develop later are IgG antibodies. IgG antibodies therefore usually signal immunity to an infectious disease. Both are specific for the infection that stimulated their development and are useful in diagnosis. If the antibodies are of the IgM type, the infection is acute; if they are of the IgG type, it is either chronic or has been obliterated, and the patient is immune to repeat infection.

Both kinds of lymphocytes release substances called cytokines, which carry messages between leukocytes and are, logically, called interleukins (IL). In this system, there is always one set that causes the signs of infection and an opposing set that antagonizes the first set and is therefore anti-inflammatory. There are at least thirteen interleukins and more that have not been clearly characterized. They are referred to numerically as IL-1 through IL-13. IL-1, -6, -8, and -12 induce inflammation, while IL-4, -10, -11, and -13 are anti-inflammatory. IL-14 through -18 have not yet been fully identified. Another important cytokine, called tumor necrosis factor-alpha (TNF-α), causes death of injured cells (and sometimes normal cells).

Prostaglandins are also cytokines and also of two types; one is proinflammatory, while the second tends to control or limit the actions of the first (anti-inflammatory). Cytokines produce specific effects in the cells to which they bind, but some, such as TNF-α, also cause fever and loss of appetite. Cytokines are produced by virtually any cell if the body is injured.

Cell membrane injury allows fluid to enter the cell by osmosis with resulting swelling (edema). The inflammatory reaction to injury not only controls the causes but cleans up after it; in the process, some normal cells are also destroyed. The signs and symptoms of what we call an infectious disease are a combination of the infection and efforts of the immune system to obliterate the infection.

Since viruses live and reproduce within cells which they do not kill, including those of viral hepatitis, it appears that the infected cell must be destroyed by the immune reaction for the virus to be eliminated. Fortunately, the body produces new, uninfected cells at a rapid rate. A significant portion of damage at the site of battle is, in fact, caused by cytokines. Damage in most tissues, if it is prolonged (chronic), is marked by scarring (fibrosis). Fibrous tissue is made up of a protein called collagen. Collagen in the liver is secreted by cells normally present called Ito or stellate cells. The functions of the stellate cells are not entirely known; we do know that they store vitamin A and do not produce collagen until they are changed by some undefined stimulus within the inflammatory process. When scarring or fibrosis in the liver is extensive, it is called cirrhosis (see chapter 2). Collagen is degraded slowly if at all and is therefore permanent.

The causes of hepatitis are legion. Each kind, whether viral or nonviral, has its own characteristics and natural history. Because viral hepatitis is transmissible to others, people are generally most concerned about its cause. Viruses that primarily damage the liver are referred to as hepatotrophic viruses (see table 5.2). This is not to say that these viruses are not found elsewhere in the body or that their damage is always confined to the liver, but their usual and primary target is the liver cell. Hepatotrophic viruses primarily attack the liver because they have protein structures on their surfaces that preferentially attach, somewhat like a lock and key, to unique protein structures on the surfaces of liver cells called receptors. Following attachment, the virus is internalized into liver cells by mechanisms that are incompletely known. Because cells other than those of the liver have similar but structurally different receptors, some of these viruses can infect other organs to a limited extent. There are seven known hepatotrophic viruses, designated A, B, C, D, E, G, and TTV (transfusion transmitted virus). The letter F was assigned to what was initially believed to be a hepatotrophic virus but turned out not to be. Viruses G and TTV, although they are hepatotrophic, have not been found to have much effect on the liver. In addition, cases of hepatitis continue to appear that are not caused by any known virus. These have been referred to as non-A-E hepatitis.

Other viruses that are not primarily hepatotrophic, such as herpes simplex, infect the liver in addition to other tissues. These will be mentioned in the following chapters. Although viruses cause by far the largest number of cases of acute hepatitis, there are more nonviral causes than viral. The most prominent of these will be discussed in chapter 6.

2. What Happens When You Have Hepatitis?

Symptoms of acute hepatitis are similar regardless of the cause. Symptoms in chronic hepatitis are often completely absent or minor and are easily ignored unless liver damage has progressed to an irreversible stage. In the majority of cases of acute viral hepatitis there are no signs and few symptoms, so that the individual is unaware that infection has occurred. Antibodies against viral hepatitis, indicating previous exposure to one of these viruses, are common in healthy people who have no recollection of ever having had an illness that might have been hepatitis. Minor symptoms are dismissed as being those of a cold or something like it. In epidemics of "infectious hepatitis," or hepatitis A (see chapter 3), as opposed to the isolated, or sporadic, case, a much greater percentage of those infected have symptoms, perhaps because the amount of virus taken in tends to be greater than in isolated cases.

Symptoms in nonviral hepatitis are similarly often vague, and the problem may go undetected unless liver tests are done. If due to drugs, symptoms disappear over time after the drug is discontinued.

Signs and Symptoms of Acute Viral Hepatitis

The first symptom of acute hepatitis is loss of appetite (anorexia), followed within a few days by nausea that may progress to vomiting. These symptoms always appear in that order but may occur so rapidly that anorexia may not be recognized as having been present before nausea. Young children may not complain of nausea before they vomit, as any parent can testify. If vomiting occurs, it usually disappears after the first few days, although nausea may persist for one to six weeks. In a few, vomiting can be so prolonged as to cause dehydration and require the administering of intravenous (IV) fluids. Mild fever, joint pains, muscle aches, and skin rash may also occur but are not usually prominent. Since nausea and vomiting are common symptoms of a number of self-limited diseases, especially in children, they are often ignored in hepatitis until the eyes turn yellow (jaundice).

An infected person's urine turns dark brown, but this also frequently goes unnoticed until the eyes have turned yellow. The color (resembling that of dark tea) comes from bilirubin that is removed from serum by the kidneys and excreted in urine. Also, because the sick liver cannot make as much bile as usual, the stool becomes very light in color. As the liver recovers, dark urine and light-colored stools disappear before the jaundice goes away.

The next sign to appear is jaundice, also called icterus (Greek for jaundice). While total serum bilirubin level, made up of bilirubin both processed and not yet processed by the liver, is less than 1.2 mg/dL, jaundice cannot be seen until levels above 3 mg/dL are reached. Levels of 30 mg/dL or even more are not uncommon in acute hepatitis, especially in those cases caused by problems other than viral infections. Bilirubin is a normal waste product (see chapter 1). It is removed from the body when it is taken up by the liver, processed, and secreted into bile. The sick liver can perform none of these steps normally. Bilirubin therefore accumulates in blood and saturates body tissues, giving them a yellowish color. It is most easily visible in the white portion of the eyes but can also be seen in the skin. Jaundice is a hard sign to ignore and is usually the reason patients are seen by a physician.

Some patients will transiently experience an irritating itching of the skin, a result of the accumulation of bile there. In smokers, distaste for cigarettes is a prominent feature. Nonsmokers often complain of a foul taste in the mouth.

As hepatitis resolves, symptoms leave in an order that is the reverse of the one in which they came—vomiting stops (usually early on), then nausea and anorexia disappear. Patients will sometimes rather abruptly realize that they are hungry again; although they may not want much, food tastes good again and does not bring on nausea. It is interesting and perhaps not surprising that starches and sweets are much better tolerated than fatty foods or meats. When appetite returns, recovery is on the way, even though the abnormal liver tests may not yet show much, if any, improvement.

Signs disappear in the order in which they came—dark urine and light-colored stools disappear at about the same time the appetite comes back. The recovering liver is again able to take up, process, and eliminate bilirubin by way of bile. It takes longer for jaundice to disappear, because bilirubin saturates tissues and must be absorbed into the blood before it can be transported to the liver. Further, bilirubin in the blood eventually becomes tightly bound to serum proteins. The liver cannot take up bilirubin that is protein-bound. Protein-bound bilirubin must first be metabolized by other tissues, a process that releases bilirubin to be removed by the liver.

Complications of Acute Viral Hepatitis

Severe and Prolonged Vomiting; Dehydration

While vomiting is common early in the course of hepatitis, it is usually short-lived (one to three days). In exceptional cases, it may be prolonged and severe. Fluids, stomach acid, and electrolytes (such as sodium, chloride, potassium) are lost with vomiting, and, since intake is severely curtailed, replacement of these through eating and drinking may be inadequate. The normal protective control mechanisms of the body guard blood volume at the expense of all else. Water in tissue freely moves into and out of blood. If a normal amount of water is not present in tissues, the total volume of blood is also less than normal, and all its components are more concentrated. If blood volume is sharply reduced, the supply of blood to tissues tends to be reduced also. When the total amount of water in the body is below normal, dehydration is present. If electrolyte concentrations (such as sodium and potassium) become abnormal, cell function is inhibited. Further, loss of stomach acid from vomiting, if severe, results in an abnormal balance between body acids and bases that result in abnormal cell function. Fortunately, the body has efficient mechanisms that correct or compensate for these problems in most circumstances, but these protective mechanisms are limited.

Severe dehydration poses several risks, including extreme electrolyte disturbance, acid-base imbalance, shock, heart irregularities, coma, cardiac arrest, and death. Blood becomes more concentrated when fluid is lost, resulting in a more viscous substance that can clot within blood vessels. Older people are more likely to have arteriosclerosis with narrowed vessels, and are consequently more likely to have problems with this viscous fluid; heart attacks or strokes may occur. Regardless of a person's age, damage may be done to the collecting tubules of the kidneys resulting from low blood supply and electrolyte disturbances. This is a type of renal failure called acute tubular necrosis, and complete recovery is possible if the underlying problem is quickly corrected. Such a complication may require that an artificial kidney be used until the patient's own kidneys recover.

For all these reasons, early treatment to prevent complications is mandatory. Vomiting can usually be controlled with antiemetic drugs. The treatment of dehydration is simple—fluids containing electrolytes are given slowly through a vein, usually in a hospital or clinic setting in case the needle comes out of the vein and has to be reinserted. Early and adequate replacement of fluid and electrolytes prevents complications in the large majority of instances.

Hepatorenal Syndrome

In very severe liver disease, most often chronic rather than acute, the kidneys may spontaneously and mysteriously fail—that is, without the presence of dehydration or electrolyte disturbances. Since the kidneys remove waste nitrogen from blood in the form of urea and assist in regulating normal electrolyte balance, urea accumulates, and imbalance of electrolytes occurs. Urea is measured by determining the levels of blood urea nitrogen (BUN). In addition, creatinine, the end product of protein metabolism normally cleared rapidly by the kidneys, accumulates. An elevation of blood potassium is especially dangerous, because if it gets high enough, the electrical rhythm of the heart fails and the heart stops beating. A markedly elevated potassium level is a hallmark of the hepatorenal syndrome and requires immediate treatment. Certain drugs can lower the potassium level but do not correct the underlying problem. Hepatorenal syndrome is difficult to correct with IV fluids or even with an artificial kidney. It is usually a terminal event, meaning that liver function is unlikely to return despite the best of treatment.

The cause or causes of hepatorenal syndrome and what triggers it are unknown. Fortunately, it occurs uncommonly and only with severe liver dysfunction. Kidneys from patients who die with this syndrome can be transplanted to a patient with a normal liver and function perfectly. The kidneys in hepatorenal syndrome are therefore normal but function improperly (a condition called functional renal failure) under the influence of some unknown substance or substances, the source of which is also unknown.

Bleeding

If the prothrombin time (see chapter 1) is severely prolonged, reflecting an inability of the liver to make it, bleeding may occur spontaneously at any place in the body. Patients under the metabolic stress of a severe illness commonly develop acute ulceration of the gastrointestinal tract, referred to, logically, as stress ulcers. Bleeding from such ulcers can be severe in any circumstance and massive if the level of prothrombin is significantly depressed. In rare cases of acute hepatitis, dilated veins in the esophagus, called esophageal varices (see the discussion of cirrhosis below), develop and sometimes rupture with massive hemorrhage.

Fulminant Hepatitis (Acute Liver Failure) and Encephalopathy

Fortunately uncommon, acute liver failure is the most devastating complication of acute hepatitis of any cause. It becomes manifest in the first week in about 50 percent of patients and in 90 percent during the first four weeks following the onset of disease. Occasionally it develops after one to three months of illness. It is rarely seen after this interval. By convention, the term "fulminant hepatitis" is usually reserved for viral hepatitis but can be used with any form of severe acute liver injury. Fulminant hepatic failure may develop extremely rapidly, with death occurring only several hours or days after the first appearance of symptoms and sometimes even before jaundice has had a chance to develop. Most if not all hepatic cells are dead or too injured to carry on the myriad functions of this vital organ, and replacement of hepatic cells by regeneration progresses too slowly to adequately keep up with cell destruction. A very prolonged prothrombin time, reflecting a low blood level of prothrombin, is the first and most reliable indication that fulminant hepatitis is present or developing. This occurs before other liver tests are markedly abnormal and can be determined as soon as symptoms bring the patient to the physician. Prothrombin concentration is a commonly used liver test that is prognostic. Normal or near-normal levels early in the illness indicate that the patient will overcome the disease in due course, while very low levels indicate a poor immediate prognosis. Intense jaundice or pronounced elevations of the serum enzymes ALT and AST do not reliably indicate a bad outcome. Low glucose levels, indicating an inability of the liver to make, and convert glycogen to, glucose and to release it into the blood also indicate a poor prognosis.

When there is a severe loss of hepatic function, the brain also does not function properly. Certain waste products of the body usually removed by the liver accumulate and interfere with normal brain function. Impairment of brain function is reflected in progressively poor mental alertness, confusion, and, finally, complete coma. This is called encephalopathy. There are many causes of encephalopathy, but, when it occurs as a complication of liver disease, it is referred to specifically as hepatic encephalopathy.

One waste product of the body is ammonia (see chapter I), which can be measured in most hospital laboratories. Although hepatic encephalopathy is a much more complicated condition than if it were simply an elevated blood ammonia level, this is a convenient marker. The higher the blood ammonia, the more the brain function is impaired. However, there are many causes of mental confusion or even coma in very ill patients, some of whom have abnormal liver tests caused by problems other than acute inflammation of the liver. Thus, it is often difficult to discern the cause of encephalopathy in those who are severely ill.

The clinical manifestations of hepatic encephalopathy are divided into four stages of increasing severity. In stage I, the abnormalities are subtle and often go undetected unless specifically searched for. Sleep patterns may become reversed, so that a person sleeps during the day but not at night. Impairment of intellectual function, such as difficulty with mental arithmetic or logical conclusions, occurs. Changes in behavior patterns often take place, although these may consist of nothing more than unusual euphoria or irritability.

Stage II is marked by some or all of the following: lethargy, amnesia, loss of a sense of time, grossly impaired ability to perform calculations, an overt change in personality, inappropriate behavior (such as using the sink as a urinal), and slurred speech. Some muscular incoordination is present, marked by the patient's inability to maintain a sustained muscle contraction. This is demonstrated by asking the person to put an arm out horizontally, with wrist extended and fingers pointed to the ceiling, and to maintain this position. The constant contraction of the muscles necessary to do so cannot be sustained by the patient with hepatic encephalopathy. The hand involuntarily and suddenly "flaps" forward and then returns to its original position. This is known as asterixis.

Patients in stage III are confused, disoriented as to time and place, given to bizarre behavior such as anger, paranoia, or rage, and have muscle function so uncoordinated that they cannot sit or walk without help. They are often stuporous but do respond to voice and painful stimuli.

Stage IV encephalopathy is marked by unconsciousness and lack of response to painful stimuli. Recovery from stage IV is rare in patients with acute hepatitis but may occur in people with chronic liver disease if it was precipitated by correctable causes such as electrolyte abnormalities or meat ingestion from which ammonia was generated by colon bacteria.

Hepatic encephalopathy is treated by restriction of dietary protein, from which ammonia is generated, and by antibiotics that inhibit the metabolism of bacteria in the colon, also a source of blood ammonia.

Swelling (edema) of the brain is a severe complication of acute hepatitis from which recovery is uncommon even with the best of treatment. Since the brain is encased in a close-fitting box of rigid bone, little space is available for enlargement. Swelling therefore results in increased pressure in this box. The only area in which the brain can expand is at the base of the skull where the spinal cord exits into the canal of the vertebrae. When the soft and swollen brain is forced or "herniates" into this small opening in response to the pressure, it is compressed, and the area that controls respiration cannot function, leading to cessation of breathing. Further, as swelling increases, the pressure in the brain exceeds blood pressure, so that blood flow to the brain slows and finally stops, leading to brain death from which there is no recovery.

Hepatic encephalopathy in acute hepatitis carries a grave prognosis but can be interrupted anywhere in its progression if recovery from the acute hepatitis occurs. Such a reversal of the course with resulting complete recovery takes place in about 50 to 60 percent of children and about 30 to 40 percent of young adults but in less than 15 percent of adults older than forty. If encephalopathy is clearly present, it means that liver damage is very severe, recovery is questionable, and arrangements for an emergency liver transplant should be made if feasible. (Research is currently being done on the creation of an artificial liver; see chapter 7.) If a person recovers from acute fulminant hepatitis, the liver is completely normal. Cirrhosis requires persistent inflammation over time and thus does not occur as a result of the relatively short duration of acute hepatitis, regardless of how severe, if it resolves.

Signs and Symptoms of Chronic Hepatitis

Chronic hepatitis is defined as inflammation of the liver that goes on for longer than six months. It is caused by an inability of the body to rid itself of virus, a patient's failure to discontinue an injurious drug, the occurrence of spontaneously developing antibodies (autoantibodies), or other persistent factors that bring about inflammation. Hepatitis A and E never cause chronic liver disease, whereas about 5 percent of people with hepatitis B acquired in adulthood and more than 75 to 80 percent of those with hepatitis C become chronic.

Once the acute process has subsided, no signs or symptoms reliably suggest the presence of chronic inflammation of the liver. Nevertheless, the process may continue, resulting in cirrhosis. Therefore, most people do not know that they have chronic hepatitis until it is discovered when blood tests are done for whatever reason. Many will say that they have been suffering from fatigue, but this is such a common symptom in even healthy people today that it is difficult to assign blame to chronic hepatitis or any other specific disease without thorough testing. Similarly, patients will sometimes complain of intermittent pain around the general area of the liver.

Although physicians can often make a diagnosis of chronic hepatitis from laboratory studies, a liver biopsy is frequently necessary to verify that abnormal blood tests are, in fact, due to chronic hepatitis. Examination of liver tissue under the microscope allows an estimation of both the amount of inflammation present and the extent of damage at the moment of the procedure. The recommendation is often made, therefore, to evaluate the effects of therapy and the progress of the disease since the last biopsy or to give some estimate of the prognosis. While a biopsy can be obtained during a surgical exploration of the abdomen, it can also be done through the skin by introducing a special needle into the liver after local anesthesia of the skin with xylocaine. Sedation or anesthesia is not required but is used in special circumstances. It is a relatively painless procedure and sometimes done under x-ray or ultrasound guidance. Just as a hollow pipe will fill with mud if pushed into wet clay, the needle fills with liver tissue.

There is commonly some mild pain at the site of the biopsy immediately afterwards, but this usually subsides within minutes. Narcotics such as Demerol are occasionally necessary. This discomfort is commonly referred to the top of the right shoulder but does not suggest a serious complication. It results from penetration of the diaphragm by the biopsy needle on its way to the liver, a common and unimportant occurrence. (Pain in the diaphragm is characteristically referred to the shoulder because of the arrangement of nerves that innervate the diaphragm.) The major risk of a liver biopsy is bleeding, but this occurs in fewer than one in two hundred procedures and is rarely fatal. The gallbladder can be in an unusual position and may be punctured by the needle, even in the hands of those with a great deal of experience. If this occurs, an emergency operation is sometimes necessary to stop the leaking of bile from the gallbladder. Of course, puncture of the lung or other organs, infection, a patient fainting or experiencing unusually severe pain, or other complications can occur. Millions of liver biopsies have been done through the skin without complications; death results in fewer than one in ten thousand procedures.

Complications of Chronic Hepatitis

Chronic inflammation causes scarring (fibrosis). Only if fibrosis becomes extensive is it called cirrhosis. Although the diagnosis of cirrhosis can sometimes be made by laboratory tests in combination with the physical examination, it must be confirmed by examination of liver tissue under the microscope. As with any scar, once present, cirrhosis remains for the life of the individual. Cirrhosis is not cancer. We cannot make scarring disappear, although there is reason to believe that it may be possible to do so in the distant future. Inflammation must be prolonged before fibrosis develops. Short-lived inflammation, as in acute hepatitis, does not cause significant fibrosis. If the inflammatory process that caused the fibrosis has been overcome, we call the cirrhosis "inactive," and liver tests are normal. If it is ongoing and producing more fibrosis—that is, adding to the cirrhosis already present—it is referred to as "active cirrhosis," and liver tests are abnormal.

Just as there are many causes of chronic inflammation of the liver, there are many causes of cirrhosis. Although the popular notion is that most people who have cirrhosis have consumed excessive amounts of alcohol, such a circumstance accounts for only a small fraction of all cases. Another widespread misconception is that everyone who has cirrhosis will inevitably die because of it. Cirrhosis is not uncommon in people who are apparently healthy. According to autopsies done on healthy adult patients in the United States who die in auto accidents, more than one in ten have unsuspected cirrhosis, having had no signs or symptoms to suggest that it was present. A rough estimate is that about half of those with cirrhosis never have signs or symptoms of the disease and may die with it but not because of it. As already noted, the liver's reserve capacity makes it able to compensate for a considerable loss of liver cells.

Edema and Ascites

When cirrhosis is present (and to a much lesser degree during acute hepatitis), there is increased resistance to the free flow of blood in the portal vein, including its final small divisions, the sinusoids. Resistance causes an increase in pressure that is transmitted along the length of the portal vein and all the veins that empty into it, including the splenic vein which drains blood from the spleen. This is referred to as portal hypertension. One can imagine what is happening by visualizing the crimping of a garden hose that is carrying water. If the flow of water is obstructed, the pressure in the hose increases and is reflected throughout the length of the hose. The increased pressure in the liver sinusoids forces water and small proteins in blood into the adjacent space that surrounds all sinusoids, called the space of Disse. This excess fluid exceeds what can be handled by the normal system of hepatic lymphatic vessels and eventually weeps from the surface of the liver. If the amount is more than can be absorbed by the lining of the abdomen, it accumulates there and is called ascites. Since this accumulation comes from the circulation and can amount to several quarts or even gallons, blood volume tends to be reduced. With this fall in blood volume the normal compensating mechanisms of the kidney begin to conserve water (which requires conservation of sodium) to keep the blood volume at a near-normal level.

A second postulated mechanism involves retention of salt and water by the kidneys before there is any fall in blood volume. This retention causes an increase in blood volume. The excess water is redistributed to body tissues and is excreted into the peritoneal cavity, causing edema and ascites, respectively. In both these mechanisms, portal hypertension is present.

There are many causes of ascites by other mechanisms and other diseases, but these are not germane to liver disease and will not be discussed here.

Serum albumin helps to keep water within blood vessels by osmosis. Low levels of albumin in blood may result in the leakage of water from blood vessels into the surrounding tissue, causing edema. Edema due to low serum albumin is most prominent in lower portions of the body, where the force of gravity adds to the tendency of fluid to leak into tissue. This means that in the upright posture, the feet and lower legs swell. Edema is not injurious and is readily reversed if the circumstance leading to it is stopped, but its presence reflects the severity of the liver disease.

Since the excess water of ascites or edema comes from protective absorption by the kidneys, and since this requires sodium, restriction of sodium in the diet (principally as table salt) will greatly reduce the amount of water absorbed and thus the amount of ascites or edema present.

A normal function of the spleen is to remove old or damaged red blood cells, white blood cells, and platelets from the circulation. In addition, the spleen stores blood cells. In portal hypertension, pressure is reflected into all veins directly connected to the portal vein. This includes the splenic vein. The spleen becomes enlarged from engorgement with blood and tends to be overly zealous, removing even normal blood cells. The result is low levels of red blood cells, white blood cells, and platelets. This is called hypersplenism.

Portal Hypertension and Bleeding Esophageal Varices

The law of fluid dynamics states that a flowing liquid will
find the path of least resistance. When blood that normally
goes through the liver and into the heart meets resistance, it
will find an easier path. One such path is to the small veins
in the esophagus that are connected to the portal system
below the diaphragm (fig. 2.1). These veins normally carry
blood from the esophagus into the portal system but now
carry blood from the portal system back to the heart. Because
the esophageal veins are carrying a much greater volume
of blood than usual and are under increased pressure, they
become large, tortuous, and thin-walled. These are called
esophageal varices and are common in cirrhosis but unusual
in acute hepatitis. When seen through an endoscope, they
look a lot like varicose veins of the legs. (An endoscope is

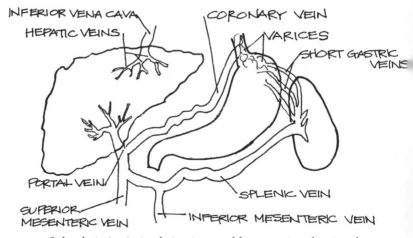

FIG. 2.1. Splanchnic (gut) circulation in portal hypertension showing the
connection between the portal vein and esophageal veins via the coronary vein.
When blood meets resistance to flow in a scarred liver, pressure is increased
in the portal vein, and this pressure is transmitted to all veins connected to
it. Thus, the normally small veins of the esophagus become varicose veins, or
varices.

a long, flexible, rubber-like solid instrument with a light-sensitive microchip on the end that transmits a picture to a video screen, allowing the inside of the tube of the gut to be seen in detail.) Unfortunately, varices are covered only by the thin inner lining of the esophagus instead of by tough skin. If the pressure in the portal vein system is high enough and if the varices become very large, they may rupture and cause life-threatening hemorrhage.

Interestingly, it is estimated that only about one-third of patients with esophageal varices will ever bleed from them. Bleeding can usually be controlled with an endoscope; rubber bands are placed around the bleeding point or the veins injected with solutions that cause clotting. Rebleeding is prevented by the repeating of one of these procedures until all visible varices are obliterated. Drugs that cause a modest reduction in portal pressure also help control bleeding varices. If these maneuvers are not successful, the portal vein can be surgically connected to the low pressure inferior vena cava, the major vein draining the legs, resulting in decreased pressure in the portal system. This operation is referred to as a portal shunt. The connection between the high pressure portal vein and the low pressure hepatic vein can be also be accomplished by introducing a long catheter equipped with a needle through a vein in the patient's neck, advancing it into the liver, through the organ's substance, and thence into a branch of the portal vein. The connection is held open by placing a wire mesh tube between the outflow vein of the liver (the hepatic vein) and the portal vein within the liver itself. This is done by radiologists and is called a transcutaneous intrahepatic portal shunt, or TIPS. Both TIPS and surgically created portal shunts are very effective in preventing further bleeding.

Fortunately, bleeding varices is a rare occurrence in acute hepatitis. If it occurs, it is usually a reason to consider an emergency liver transplant.

Cancer of the Liver

Cancer that begins in the liver is an important health problem, and its frequency has increased throughout the world. In 1990 it ranked fifth as the cause of known cancer deaths in the United States, with 427,000 cases reported. The majority of cases have well-established cirrhosis at the time of discovery. There are two types: hepatocellular carcinoma from liver cells and cholangiolar carcinoma from bile ducts. Although cirrhosis may be of any kind, both hepatitis B and C have been strongly implicated as predisposing causes of hepatocellular carcinoma. The frequency of hepatocellular carcinoma varies from as much as 20 percent in those with a twenty-year history of chronic hepatitis C and cirrhosis in Asia (where 76 percent of all cases are found) to about 5 percent of these cases in the United States. The increase in frequency due to chronic hepatitis B is similar. To be sure, there are other factors associated with cancer of the liver. Chief among these are aflatoxins, products of the fungus *Aspergillus flavus*, a ubiquitous contaminant of virtually all foods whether commercially or privately produced.

Signs of Cirrhosis

Signs that suggest the possible presence of cirrhosis include an enlarged spleen, ascites, and edema of the feet and legs. The liver size may be smaller than normal if it has shrunk from disease or large if the causative inflammation is still present. Jaundice is usually not present unless cirrhosis is in its terminal phase or inflammation is still present. Occasionally, bleeding from esophageal varices is the first sign that portal hypertension is present and may occur with little other evidence of cirrhosis. Encephalopathy may herald cirrhosis, but other signs are usually present. In long-established cirrhosis with portal hypertension, connections develop between the portal vein and the veins around the umbilicus (the "belly button"). These veins are the remnants of the umbilical vein, the vessel that supplied blood to the fetus from the mother. This connection allows blood to flow from the portal vein back to the heart by going around the scarred liver. These sometimes have the appearance of a mass of vessels and are called caput medusae, in reference to the mythological Greek character who had snakes for hair.

Because of certain hormonal abnormalities in cirrhosis not discussed here, male patients with cirrhosis will often develop enlargement of their breasts (gynecomastia) as well as atrophy (shrinkage) of the testicles. Others will develop connections between arterioles and veins in the skin referred to as "hepatic spiders," which are more accurately called hepatic arteriovenous malformations. This direct transfer of arterial pressure into veins with less pressure causes the formation of a central point that pulsates with each beat of the heart. Seeing this pulsation requires special effort. With the naked eye, one can see vessels branching away from the central point, giving the appearance of a spider. Single hepatic spiders can be seen in healthy young persons, most commonly in women of childbearing age, but, if numerous, are reliable signs that cirrhosis is present.

3. Hepatitis A

Prevalence

Epidemics of hepatitis A are not just ancient history—they continue to occur. Worldwide, over 1,000,000 cases of hepatitis with jaundice are reported every year. In the United States, where the frequency of infection is lower than in many other countries, there are some 140,000 recognized cases each year, the majority of which are isolated ones with no recognized exposure. Outbreaks continue to occur because the virus is present in the population even when the disease is not made apparent by jaundice. Within the past few years, an epidemic of over 1,000 cases occurred in an outbreak in Memphis, Tennessee, and another with over 500 cases in northern California. A 1988 epidemic in China involved 200,000 to 300,000 cases.

The actual number of infections is difficult to estimate because the majority of people affected are asymptomatic, do not become jaundiced, and therefore go undiagnosed. Such individuals serve as a reservoir of the virus and source of infection for others. The actual rate of infection must be judged by the presence of antibodies against hepatitis A, indicating exposure to the virus even if jaundice has not occurred. In the United States, depending on the socioeconomic group studied, from about 10 percent of children younger than five years old to 75 percent of adults over fifty have antibodies. Overall, between 40 and 45 percent of the U.S. population have antibodies against hepatitis A. According to these data, over 100,000,000 people now living in the United States have been infected at some time in the past. In countries with poor public sanitation, up to 90 perecent of all adults have evidence of past infection. Clearly, the virus is always with us.

The Virus

By the end of the 1940s, it was recognized that there were at least two types of hepatitis based on differences in the time it took for illness to appear after a known exposure. This is called the incubation period. These two varieties were called infectious or short incubation hepatitis and serum or long incubation hepatitis (see table 5.2). Research on volunteers and at institutions in which hepatitis was endemic proved that the short incubation infectious agent was present in feces of those ill with the disease and that the incubation period was two to six weeks. It was labeled MS-1 (infectious hepatitis). The second was shown to be transmitted by blood and body secretions and to have an incubation period of one to two months; it was labeled MS-2 (serum hepatitis). The virus causing infectious hepatitis was observed by electron microscopy in feces in 1973 and thereafter was known as hepatitis A virus (HAV) (fig. 3.1). Logically, the virus of serum hepatitis was called hepatitis B virus (HBV).

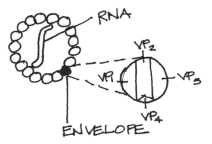

FIG. 3.1. Structure of the hepatitis A virus. VP1, VP2, VP3, and VP4 are the four proteins of the envelope that are produced under the direction of the P1 portion of the gene (see fig. 3.2).

By the 1960s, we had learned how to culture living animal and human tissue cells in laboratory dishes. Since all viruses require living cells for growth, this accomplishment provided a medium in which viruses could be studied outside the body. Such a preparation enabled study of the structure, function, and growth characteristics of a number of viruses, including HAV, HBV, and polio. Interestingly, it takes from one to four months for all the cells in a culture to become infected with HAV after inoculation of the culture medium, whereas it takes only two to six weeks after infection for people to become ill.

The genetic material of all the hepatotrophic viruses is ribonucleic acid (RNA), except for hepatitis B, in which case it is deoxyribonucleic acid (DNA). Nucleic acids are the fundamental substances of all living things and are so named because they were first isolated from cell nuclei. They are present in nuclei as genes that pass on the heredity character-istics of the organism. They are also present in the cytoplasm of the cell, where they cause the manufacture of all proteins characteristic of the species. (Thus frog cells make more frog cells and frog proteins.) The genes of viruses and bacteria be-have similarly. The two classes of nucleic acids are ribonucleic acid (RNA) and deoxyribonucleic acid (DNA). In the form of coiled, or helical, strands, these constitute the backbone of the gene, and each has thousands of molecules of amino acids attached. The sequence of the amino acids determines the structure of protein that is made or the characteristics of the genes that result from replication of the cells.

The only natural host for HAV is humans. Only cell cul-tures from humans and from a few nonhuman primates (mar-mosets and chimpanzees) support its growth. The single gene of hepatitis A is a strand of RNA (fig. 3.2). We can identify three main segments of the gene, called P1, P2, and P3. Although these segments vary among hepatitis A viruses isolated from different parts of the world, there is 75 to 90 percent similarity, so that the single antibody generated by the presence of any strain is highly effective against all strains.

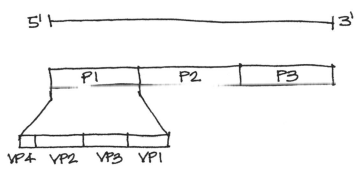

FIG. 3.2. Genome of the single strand of RNA that is the gene of the hepatitis A virus. The orientation of genes is conventionally marked at one end with a 5'designation (indicating the chemical structure of a specific protein) and at the other end by a 3'protein. These regions are not translated, meaning that they do not cause any protein production. The gene has only three divisions—P1, P2, and P3.

Thus, the vaccine that stimulates antibody against hepatitis A is effective against all strains.

There is no evidence that the presence of the virus in the cell causes its death. In cell cultures, no damage to the cells occurs unless serum containing antibodies and white blood cells is added to the culture media, whereupon infected cells and the virus they contain are promptly destroyed.

HAV is resistant to the acid environment of the stomach. It also survives heat exposure at 60°C (140°F) for sixty minutes but is inactivated at 85°C (185°F) for one minute. Thus, cooking destroys HAV and is important in the prevention of its transmission. The virus can survive in sea water for an unknown period, in feces at room temperature for four weeks, and in live oysters for five days.

The Disease

Transmission of HAV occurs by the fecal-oral route in person-to-person contact. As discussed above, the virus is present in feces from infected persons, most of whom are not ill. Infants and children younger than two years of age who are infected are rarely sick but shed great numbers of virus in their stools. This age group is, of course, the one most likely to cause contamination of their environment with feces. Colon bacteria from healthy people can be cultured from almost any surface, and, where these bacteria are present, any associated virus is also present. Thus, when hepatitis A is around, it passes easily from one person to another unless stringent precautions are taken. When many people are infected, as in an epidemic, more of the virus is around, which makes it more likely that additional people will become infected. Infected people who recover develop antibodies and are thereafter immune. Epidemics continue until there are no more susceptible people to become infected or until steps are taken to interrupt the cycle.

As one would expect, the virus is always present in any sewer system. Treatment of sewage before it is released into the oceans is generally but not totally effective in destroying HAV. There are well-documented cases in which contamination of oyster beds resulted in outbreaks of the disease. Shellfish in general and oysters in particular process large volumes of water, so that any virus present becomes concentrated. The virus is passed to susceptible hosts if these foods are consumed without having been thoroughly cooked.

The virus can be passed if a person eats contaminated food or touches a contaminated surface and then places the fingers in or about the mouth without washing the hands. Simply washing with soap and water readily destroys the virus. In one study of an epidemic, almost 15 percent of those sick with hepatitis were employees of or attended daycare centers where the changing of diapers was a daily necessity. Children, not known for their inherent cleanliness, can easily pass the virus on to other children and to their parents, even when they themselves are not ill.

The source of infection is unknown in about 40 percent of cases despite careful searching. These sources apparently are infected persons with or without illness who pass the virus to others by preparing food without careful hand washing or by close personal contact such as in sexual activities, kissing, or the sharing of eating utensils.

The person who is well but in the incubation period of the disease can pass along large amounts of virus in feces. The danger is obvious only when the individual becomes ill with hepatitis A. If this person works in a food establishment, public health officials in a community will recommend that everyone who ate in a particular place during a certain period of time get prophylactic treatment to prevent disease. (More information about prevention appears later in this chapter.)

The virus passes through the intestinal wall and appears in blood (viremia) where it can be detected for about two weeks. Thereafter, the virus can be found only in the liver, where it reproduces. After the virus is transported to the liver in the portal vein, it attaches to receptors on the surface of liver cells. After attachment, the virus is internalized, reproduces within the cytoplasm of the cell, and is excreted into bile and thence into the gut. Virus appears in feces as early as two weeks before any signs or symptoms of disease are present.

When viremia is present early in the incubation period, transmission of HAV can occur by blood exchange. This mode of transmission has been seen with increasing frequency among IV drug users in the age range of nineteen to thirty-nine. During the 1990s, drug-associated outbreaks occurred in at least five states, with numbers ranging from sixteen hundred to five thousand cases. In rare cases, hepatitis A has followed transfusion with blood obtained from such persons.

Since the symptoms of acute hepatitis are similar without regard to the cause, they are grouped together, and were discussed in chapter 2.

A common but false belief is that if the person who transmits the disease is extremely ill, it is more likely that the recipient will also be very ill. The severity of disease is a function of the host's reaction to the infection, not the virulence of the virus or the severity of the case from which the virus was transmitted. As we have seen, most cases probably originate in people who are not sick at all. Some of these new cases, of course, become quite symptomatic. It is known that a heavy infecting load of virus results in more severe disease, apparently because more hepatic cells are infected. With a greater number of infected cells, more will be destroyed by the defenses of the host. Disease severity and outcomes depend on three factors: (1) the activity of the immune system; (2) the number of infected hepatic cells; and (3) the rapidity with which destroyed hepatic cells are replaced.

It has long been observed that, for unknown reasons, the older the person is who is infected with hepatitis A, the more serious the disease will be: symptoms are more severe, complications occur more often, and the mortality rate is higher. Children younger than two have high rates of infection, but only about 15 percent become jaundiced or have notable symptoms, and they rarely die because of the disease. When it occurs in childhood or adolescence, the disease tends to be mild, although devastating complications are occasionally seen. About 75 percent of children have jaundice with the disease, but the mortality rate is less than one in ten thousand (0.01 percent). In adults older than forty years of age jaundice occurs in nearly 100 percent, and the mortality rate is close to two per one hundred (2 percent). The average mortality rate for all ages is around three per one thousand (0.3 percent)

During the incubation period, the virus is reproducing within liver cells, while the immune system, stimulated by the presence of the virus, is developing defenses. The immune system of the host has been generally accepted as the mechanism by which destruction of the virus occurs, liver tests become abnormal, and the individual becomes ill. Most of the symptoms are caused by cytokines that are released during cell destruction (see chapter 2).

Since virus is present in stools about two weeks before there is any evidence of disease and while the patient is still active and not confined to home, persons not yet ill are those most likely to pass the virus to others. Patients are also considered infectious for about one week after jaundice has appeared because the virus is still in stools during that time. Children younger than two years of age recover rapidly with a very low frequency of complications. In adults and children over six, more acute symptoms such as nausea and vomiting usually improve or disappear within about seven days, but anorexia may persist for several additional days. Patients usually feel quite well, and liver tests return to normal in two to four weeks.

There are two variant clinical forms of hepatitis A. Cholestatic hepatitis refers to an uncommon form in which there is moderate to severe generalized itching. Liver tests show unusually elevated levels of serum alkaline phosphatase (see chapter 1), suggesting a problem with secretion of bile. These liver tests resemble ones obtained in patients with obstruction of bile flow and may cause confusion in diagnosis. Cholestatic hepatitis A also tends to be associated with symptoms for somewhat longer than the usual form (ten to twelve weeks), but its prognosis for complete recovery is good.

Relapsing hepatitis, the second variant form, is also uncommon. It is characterized by two or more bouts of acute symptoms occurring over a six-to-ten-week period. The total serum bilirubin and liver enzyme (ALT and AST) concentrations may appear to be rapidly falling towards normal levels, only to see another wave of abnormal liver tests and jaundice. It has the same good prognosis as the more common form.

It is important to know that hepatitis A does not cause chronic hepatitis and therefore never leads to cirrhosis, regardless of the severity of the acute disease. Furthermore, it never lasts longer than six months. It has been associated with the onset of signs and symptoms of autoimmune diseases such as rheumatoid arthritis or even autoimmune liver disease.

Diagnosis

In the patient with jaundice (i.e., an elevated serum bilirubin) and characteristic symptoms, the diagnosis is not difficult. Jaundice is usually present in those recognized as having the disease. The liver is enlarged and mildly tender. The urine becomes dark and the stools light in color (see chapter 2). It is, of course, helpful to know if there has been exposure to a known case of hepatitis. Even in patients with severe symptoms, a normal prothrombin time is reliably predictive of an uneventful resolution of the disease. Conversely, a prolonged prothrombin time indicates very severe disease.

Although it is usually the appearance of jaundice that prompts a visit to a physician, serum ALT and AST become abnormal several days before jaundice is present. The first set of liver tests show serum ALT and AST levels that are elevated, usually in the range of five hundred to a thousand units/mL, but levels of thirty-five hundred are common. Interestingly, neither the ALT nor the AST goes over four thousand U/mL in viral hepatitis, but they do so frequently in nonviral hepatitis. The peak levels of these enzymes do not correlate with the severity of symptoms or predict the outcome of the disease. Indeed, patients with jaundice but with few or even no symptoms may have the same serum enzyme levels as those with severe nausea, vomiting, and lethargy. In the first seven to ten days, the ALT and AST continue to rise and thereafter fall with variable rapidity, reaching normal levels in about two to four weeks.

Biopsy of the liver is no longer considered necessary for a diagnosis except in unusual cases. When necessary, it is a safe procedure. Examination of liver tissue aids in ruling out other diseases that may have similar laboratory findings. It will confirm the inflammatory process but does not reveal the cause.

Because of differences in long-term prognosis, it is imperative to determine which of the several kinds of viral hepatitis is present. This is done by determining the presence and type of antibodies against viruses that cause hepatitis (see table 5.1). In acute hepatitis A, anti-HAV antibodies appear promptly and are present when the disease is discovered. It is important to know that the usual test for these antibodies will be reported as positive if either the acute antibody (IgM) or the immune antibody (IgG) is present. Obviously, a person who has been exposed to hepatitis A in the past and is immune can have some other form of viral hepatitis. Therefore a positive test must be followed with a test for the IgM antibody specific for the acute disease. The IgM antibody persists for several months and is gradually replaced by IgG antibody that represents immunity. It is possible to test for the RNA of HAV, but the test is expensive and done almost exclusively in research laboratories.

Management

No specific treatment will shorten the course, decrease the severity, or prevent complications of hepatitis A. Hospitalization is therefore reserved for those with complications. Acute viral hepatitis A is a self-limited disease.

Up until about forty or fifty years ago, patients with acute viral hepatitis were routinely hospitalized or confined to bed at home for weeks or months on the unfounded assumption that exertion would make the disease more severe and last longer. Patients were put to bed until jaundice disappeared and all liver tests were entirely normal. The effect of exercise on acute hepatitis has been tested in our military. One group with hepatitis was hospitalized and kept inactive, while another went on forced marches after the initial symptoms improved. When each group was evaluated some several weeks and then a few years later, recovery in the exercise group was not delayed and no long-term adverse outcomes were seen. Later studies have reinforced these observations. Since forced bed rest has certain adverse results, patients should be encouraged to do what they feel like doing. Because hospitalization exposes other patients and personnel to infection and provides no specific treatment, it is avoided in uncomplicated disease. Vitamins and purified protein diets were previously widely prescribed without scientific support and are no longer used. Nevertheless, approximately 10 to 20 percent of patients require hospitalization, most commonly for prolonged vomiting and dehydration. Fluids given intravenously can quickly and effectively replace lost fluids and prevent the complications of dehydration.

Medications to control vomiting are variably helpful. Unfortunately, some antiemetics occasionally cause abnormal liver tests, and many physicians are afraid to use them in patients with acute hepatitis. However, these patients are no more (and no less) likely to have adverse liver reactions than those without liver disease.

Nausea and lack of appetite result in a patient's having little or no food intake early in the disease. Drinking fluids to prevent dehydration is much more important than food intake, at least in the first several days of illness. Fluids are generally well tolerated, especially carbonated drinks. Ingestion of small amounts (one or two swallows) every fifteen to twenty minutes provides as much as one liter (about one quart) of fluid per day, quite enough to avoid dehydration. Intense nausea usually disappears within two to seven days, and, although anorexia persists for several days thereafter, small amounts of food can be consumed without provoking more vomiting. Frequent feedings of small portions are often well tolerated. Forcing food on a patient during the early days of hepatitis tends to make nausea and vomiting worse. As soon as appetite returns, a normal diet is advised. In those who were healthy before the disease, this brief period of inadequate food intake is not harmful. Meat and especially fatty foods are particularly repulsive to a patient with nausea from almost any cause.

Patients who have profound and persistent nausea lasting longer than seven to ten days may require hospitalization for intravenous feedings of calories in the form of elemental sugars, amino acids, and fatty acids. It is now commonplace to use such feedings to completely supply all nutritional requirements indefinitely in patients who cannot eat for whatever reason.

Prevention

Good personal hygiene and public sanitation facilities inhibit the spread of hepatitis A but will not prevent all cases, given the ubiquitous presence of the virus in the environment. People who have been exposed are advised to get injections of gamma globulin, which contains antibodies against hepatitis A. This preparation is made from the pooled globulin fraction of serum from the general population and treated to kill all living organisms. Given that some 40 percent of our population have antibodies against HAV, this provides concentrated antibodies that prevent infection immediately and for about four months thereafter. The most common situation in which such prophylaxis is indicated pertains to family members of someone with an acute case. Since the virus is present in feces for at least two weeks before jaundice occurs, family members will have already been exposed when the acute case is discovered. The injections are highly effective (at least 98 percent) if given within two to three days of exposure, but less so if more time elapses, and they are ineffective if given two weeks after exposure, because the antibodies given are destroyed by the body's metabolism and not replaced until the immune system is able to respond to the infection. The recommended dose is 0.02 mL gamma globulin for each kilogram of body weight of the exposed person. (A kilogram is 2.2 pounds.) Gamma globulin injections are locally painful and can cause fever and muscle aches for a few days.

There are two licensed vaccines made of virus grown in cell culture and then killed. Both induce the development of antibodies against HAV but require about three weeks to do so. Both are highly effective in inducing immunity to HAV and preventing the disease. Large groups at risk for acute hepatitis A have been shown to be 98 to 100 percent protected. The recommended dose of each is 1 mL in adults and ½ mL in children, followed in six to twelve months by a second dose. Neither is licensed for use in children younger than two years of age. Vaccines are recommended for those at high risk of exposure, which includes travelers to areas where the diease is endemic, military personnel, the sexually promiscuous (both heterosexuals and homosexuals), health care workers, employees of daycare centers, users of illicit drugs, and workers in institutions where the disease is prevalent.

Adverse effects from these vaccines are few, but cardiovascular collapse has been known to occur in rare cases of allergy. Other adverse effects have included short-lived redness and swelling at the site of injection, low-grade fever, muscle aches, and nausea.

Vaccines for long-term protection and gamma globulin for immediate and short-term protection can be given simultaneously. Both are frequently recommended in epidemics and for exposure which is suspected but not proven (as when a food handler in a restaurant is discovered to have acute hepatitis A).

Since humans are the only known reservoir of HAV and since vaccines are so effective, it is theoretically possible to eliminate HAV by means of the same approach that was used for smallpox. However, this would be very expensive, and the universal presence of the virus makes it uncertain that such an effort would be successful.

Although controversial, some data suggest that patients with chronic hepatitis B or C fair poorly if they acquire acute hepatitis A; the vaccine is recommended for these patients as well.

4. Hepatitis B

The second hepatotrophic virus identified was serum hepatitis, MS-2, or hepatitis B. It has probably been around for as long as hepatitis A. This virus was identified in 1965 by Baruch Blumberg, who studied thousands of blood samples in his search for inherited traits in populations in different geographic areas of the world. He noted a reaction between an unknown antigen in the serum of an Australian aborigine and an antibody from a patient with hemophilia who had received multiple blood transfusions. Electron microscopy of serum from the aborigine revealed the presence of viral particles. Subsequently, a laboratory technician developed acute hepatitis while working with this preparation, confirming that the material was infectious and that it caused serum hepatitis. For several years, the viral antigens were referred to as "Australia antigen." For his work, Dr. Blumberg won the Nobel Prize in 1976. Related viruses have been identified that infect only nonhuman primates (chimpanzees), ground squirrels, woodchucks, and Peking ducks.

Hepatitis B is a more serious disease than hepatitis A because complications are more common. Some people become carriers of the virus with no symptoms or evidence of liver disease, while about 5 percent of exposed adults develop chronic hepatitis that can lead to cirrhosis and hepatocellular carcinoma.

Prevalence

About 350 million people in the world are infected with the hepatitis B virus (HBV). The number who die each year with this infection approaches 1 million. Over half the population of Southeast Asia, China, and Africa are infected at some time in their lives, and 8 percent are chronic carriers. The carrier rate varies from less than 1 percent to as much as 20 percent of different populations of the world, with lowest rates in New Zealand, Australia, Western Europe, and North America. Some geographic or ethnic groups such as Alaskan Eskimos and Australian aborigines have higher prevalence of infection than other groups living in immediate proximity. African Americans and Hispanics have higher prevalence than others in the United States. A major problem in areas with high carrier rates is transmission from a mother who is a carrier to her infant. These babies seldom have acute hepatitis, but about 90 percent become carriers of the disease and are able to transmit it to others. If the infection occurs later, between the ages of two to five years, the carrier rate is between 25 and 50 percent but only 5 percent thereafter. In the United States, some 98 percent of all babies born to mothers who are carriers are immediately immunized. Extrapolated data from population surveys suggest that about 5 percent of people in the United States have evidence of past exposure, the vast majority of whom are immune. Since 1985, the number of people who become infected annually has fallen by about 50 percent and is now estimated to be about forty per ten thousand.

The Virus (Fig. 4.1)

HBV has a viral core structure with an envelope that protects the virus against host defenses. It has four genes: S, P, C, and X (fig. 4.2). The S gene codes for surface protein (antigen) of the envelope, the P gene codes for polymerase, the C gene codes for core proteins and one called "e protein," and the X gene codes for an "X protein," the function of which is uncertain. Each of these protein-antigens stimulates the formation of antibodies by the host. The detection of antigens or of antibodies to surface and core protein is useful for

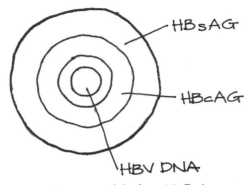

FIG. 4.1. Structure of the hepatitis B virus.
The entire particle is called the Dane particle.

diagnostic purposes (see table 5.1). Polymerase is an enzyme essential to HBV replication and is not present at other times. The function of the X protein is not fully known, but it may be an important factor in the development of hepatocellular carcinoma, which is associated with chronic HBV infection. Viruses with a mutation in the X gene cannot infect cell cultures. It therefore seems essential for replication, but its antibody is not measured except for research purposes.

Surface protein is part of the protective envelope of the virus and is referred to as hepatitis B surface antigen, or HBsAg. Since this envelope surrounds the entire virus, other elements are hidden from antibodies that develop as a response to antigens that are secreted or lost from the virus during its natural death or by other unknown means. Surface antigen is essential for survival of the virus. It is present in all acute and chronic infections, including the carrier state. Its presence therefore does not distinguish these three phases of infection. Antibodies against HBsAg are highly effective in destroying the envelope or surface of the virus. Their presence indicates that the virus has been destroyed and the patient is immune. The intact virus is referred to as the

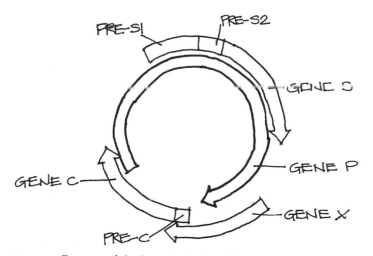

FIG. 4.2. Genome of the hepatitis B virus. The S gene is responsible for surface protein-antigen (HBsAg). The P gene is responsible for DNA polymerase, which is necessary for virus replication. The C gene is responsible for the core protein (HBcAg), while its pre-C portion is responsible for e antigen. The protein produced under the direction of the X gene (HBxAg) is uncertain.

Dane particle (see fig. 4.1). Surface protein is used to produce vaccines against HBV.

The core protein-antigen is difficult to measure in the hospital laboratory, but the antibody it stimulates (HBcAb, core antibody) is not. It is part of the usual serological tests for HBV. It becomes positive early in the acute phase and persists for years thereafter, but it is not a protective antibody because it cannot reach the core gene that is protected by the surface envelope and does not, by itself, indicate immunity. In the acute phase, core antibody is in the form of IgM globulin. About four to six months after the acute disease has been overcome, the globulin type is IgG. This difference in globulin type is useful for diagnostic purposes, since IgM globulin indicates that the cause of jaundice is acute hepatitis B.

The antibodies to hepatitis B core protein cross-react with other proteins; thus, HBcAb tests can be positive when there has been no exposure to HBV. An important example is its cross-reaction to hepatitis C protein. In various reports, between 25 and 50 percent of patients with chronic hepatitis C will have a positive hepatitis B core antibody test. In such cases, it is difficult to say that the hepatitis B core antibody is "only" a cross-reaction and not representative of previous exposure to HBV, because many hepatitis C patients acquire their disease during needle sharing, and hepatitis B may also be acquired in this way. A positive test for core antibody in the absence of other antibodies against HBV therefore calls for a test specific to hepatitis C as well as additional tests for hepatitis B. Further, no disease of any kind is found in up to 15 to 20 percent of instances of such isolated tests.

A portion of the gene called the pre-core portion codes for e antigen (HBeAg). This antigen stimulates an antibody (e antibody) that is diagnostically important because it reflects active replication of the virus. A positive test for the HBe antigen indicates that the virus is continuing to reproduce itself, while presence of the antibody indicates that it is not.

There is a form of HBV in which a mutation in the pre-core region has occurred. This form, common in parts of northern Italy but uncommon in the United States, produces all the antigens described above with the important exception of e antigen. Since it cannot produce e antigen, e antibody is not produced by the host. While the physician expects to see a positive test for the e antigen in acute viral hepatitis B, and, further, expects to see the e antibody appear as the disease is overcome, neither is present when this mutant virus is the cause of the disease. In all other respects, the mutant virus causes the same disease as does the "wild" or nonmutant virus with the same rate of complications. Vaccines are equally effective against the mutant variety because they are made against the surface antigen, not the e antigen. Related viruses that have been found in ground squirrels, woodchucks, and the Peking duck do not infect humans, but are useful for research because their behavior and response to drugs is similar to the human variety. HBV is rather easily destroyed by chlorine-containing disinfectants. It persists on exposed surfaces for only a matter of hours.

The Disease

Acute Hepatitis B

HBV can be detected in blood, semen, saliva, cervical secretions, and white blood cells. Transmission of the virus, however, has been documented only in exchange of blood. It is easily transmitted by the sharing of needles during IV drug use, snorting of cocaine with contaminated nasal straws, during childbirth, or sharing of razors. Epidemiologic data clearly indicate the possibility of transmission during sexual intercourse, not only from men to women and women to men, but also from men to men (especially anal receptive) and women to women. The use of shared toothbrushes may result in transmission of the disease, not through ingestion but through blood exchange. Other as yet unknown methods of transmission may exist. The virus is destroyed by acid in the stomach, so that ingestion of contaminated food or water or use of eating utensils after they have been used by an infected person is highly unlikely to result in transmission of the disease. Thus, household contacts (if there is no sexual exposure) do not pose a significant risk. In some 20 to 30 percent of acute cases, the mode of transmission is unknown.

HBV was commonly transmitted by blood transfusions before tests to identify the virus were developed. Donated blood is now routinely examined for HBV and transmission by transfusion is unusual. Nevertheless, about a hundred cases of documented transfusion-associated acute hepatitis B occur every year. Given the many thousands of blood transfusions annually, this is a remarkably low incidence. The appearance of AIDS has significantly changed sexual practices and has probably been responsible for further reduction in the annual attack rate. Casual social contact, such as working in an office with a person infected with HBV, is not a risk factor.

The incubation period of hepatitis B is four to sixteen weeks (see table 5.2). As noted, acute viral hepatitis may occur with no signs or symptoms. The acute illness tends to be somewhat more prolonged than that of acute hepatitis A, but the symptoms are the same in all varieties of viral hepatitis (see chapter 2). Whereas most patients with acute hepatitis A are feeling quite well in two to four weeks, most hepatitis B patients require an average of two to three months to feel recovered and to have normal energy levels. Nausea and vomiting usually subside within two to six weeks. The average time off work is about four to six weeks.

Jaundice usually does not go above a level of 5–10 mg/dL but may reach levels of 30 mg/dL. The degree of elevation does not predict the outcome, nor does it distinguish one form of liver disease from another. In acute hepatitis B, serum bilirubin levels tend to rise more slowly and reach a peak later than in hepatitis A. The peak level usually occurs in one to three weeks, falling rapidly for seven to ten days and thereafter more slowly until it reaches a normal level in three to four months. If the level of serum bilirubin is plotted against time in weeks or months, it forms a curved line with the highest portion well to the left of center—that is, early in the course. If the bilirubin curve forms a plateau and remains elevated for longer than four weeks, acute or subacute hepatic failure is a concern. The curve of bilirubin levels lags behind that of the serum enzymes ALT and AST; that is, the enzyme levels peak before that of bilirubin and reach normal levels before the bilirubin.

The ALT and AST levels are elevated when the patient is first seen. The levels reached tend to be lower than those seen in hepatitis A and do not exceed 4,000 U/dL in the uncomplicated case. The level of enzymes, like that of bilirubin, does not predict the outcome of acute hepatitis. As a rule, these enzymes begin to fall rapidly within the first two weeks and reach normal levels in one to two months.

Because hepatic cells swell when injured, bile flow in the smallest bile ducts is inhibited by compression by the cells surrounding them. Thus the alkaline phosphatase may be mildly elevated in the first several days of illness but then becomes normal. In contrast to hepatitis A, there is no cholestatic form of hepatitis B.

The prothrombin time may be prolonged one to five seconds (thirteen to seventeen seconds compared to a normal of twelve seconds). A prolongation of more than this is worrisome because of the possibility of acute liver failure and must be followed closely.

Complications of acute hepatitis B are similar to those of acute hepatitis A or C and are discussed in chapter 2. The frequency of encephalopathy and acute hepatic failure is higher in hepatitis B than in hepatitis A but is still quite uncommon. Even in large hospitals in which many cases of viral hepatitis are seen, such instances occur infrequently.

Hepatitis B Carrier State

The term "carrier state" is applied to those who are infected and may transmit HBV but do not themselves have disease signs or symptoms.

Some patients, perhaps fewer than 3 percent, are unable to obliterate the virus but manage to control it. Liver tests are persistently normal and liver biopsy shows little or no damage. HBsAg remains detectable in serum. In the usual case, e antigen is no longer present and e antibody is present, indicating no active replication of the virus. Blood of the carrier is infectious but with low probability of transmission short of donating blood for transfusion. The virus is detectable only in tissue when amplified by PCR and through the use of special techniques. In recent years, a technique has been developed and made readily available to clinicians allowing us to isolate rare specific sequences of DNA in a mixture and to multiply them billions of times in a few hours. This is known as the "polymerase chain reaction," or PCR. Since the rate of the reaction is known, the final number of DNA particles reflects the number present originally. The number of DNA particles is a direct reflection of the number of virus particles and therefore represents a count of the load of virus present in the original sample. As few as a hundred viral particles can be measured by this technique. The carrier state is permanent in the majority. Rarely, a carrier becomes immune, at which point surface antigen disappears and antibodies against surface antigen appear. The life span of the carrier is normal, although the frequency of hepatocellular carcinoma may be increased in those who have been carriers since birth. Carriers rarely respond to drug treatment against HBV, which is thus not recommended. In a few, the disease "flares," or becomes active. The e antigen is present during a flare, and liver tests become abnormal. In most cases, the disease follows a benign course, with the final result being an immune state.

Chronic Hepatitis B

While over 90 percent of adults infected with HBV overcome the disease and obliterate the virus, about 5 percent develop chronic hepatitis. With chronic inflammation, fibrosis (scarring) slowly accumulates, finally becoming profuse enough to be classified as cirrhosis. This takes around twenty years, but some cases progress more rapidly. Unfortunately, we cannot reliably predict how fast the disease is going to progress, although microscopic findings on biopsy are helpful in judging rapidity of progression. The percentage of patients with chronic disease who progress to cirrhosis is not known, but, given enough time, most probably do. Further, the frequency of hepatocellular carcinoma is increased in those with cirrhosis from any cause. Chronic hepatitis B is therefore a risk factor for developing hepatocellular carcinoma.

Chronic hepatitis B is usually fortuitously discovered. The risk of developing chronic hepatitis B rather than overcoming the infection is increased in patients with defective or inhibited immune systems. This includes those on chronic hemodialysis for renal failure, those on drugs that suppress the immune system (such as are used in chemotherapy for cancer or organ transplants), and those infected with human immunodeficiency virus (HIV). Liver biopsy is necessary to determine the amount of damage present and is often, but not always, performed in order to quantify the amount of inflammation present. This allows a prediction of the likelihood that cirrhosis will develop if no treatment is given; it is therefore prognostic.

Manifestations of hepatitis B may also occur in other organ systems. In the acute disease, skin rash is common. The first symptom may be joint pain that can precede any signs or symptoms of hepatitis by several days or even a few weeks. Acute nephritis and inflammation of blood vessels (vasculitis) of the skin are a recognized complication. Joint pain may persist into the chronic phase of the disease.

Diagnosis

Acute Hepatitis B

Because the majority of patients with acute viral hepatitis B do not become jaundiced or have symptoms, they go undiagnosed. (Signs and symptoms that are common to all forms are discussed in chapter 2.)

As in hepatitis A, there is no evidence that HBV within the liver cell causes death of the cell. A vigorous immune response, consisting of cytokines, cytotoxic ("killer") T lymphocytes, and antibodies against the proteins made by the virus, destroys the liver cells infected with the virus, killing both the cells and the virus they contain. As hepatic cells are destroyed, they are replaced. Severity of the acute disease is related to the number of infected cells, the vigor of the host immune response, and the rapidity with which injured cells are replaced. Since the vast majority of cases of acute hepatitis B go undetected and 95 percent of those who have it completely recover and are thereafter immune, it would appear that this is an efficient process.

A history of multiple sexual partners or of IV drug use in someone with acute hepatitis suggests the possibility of hepatitis B. Note again, however, that in 20 to 30 percent of cases, no risk factors can be identified. The physical examination in the acute case may reveal jaundice and a moderately enlarged, tender liver.

The diagnosis is made by serologic testing (see table 5.1). In acute hepatitis B, surface antigen (HBsAg) is present as well as antibodies to core antigen and e antigen. The antibody to core antigen is of the IgM type. Antibodies to surface antigen and e antigen are present until recovery. Since hepatitis A is so common, the individual may also be immune to HAV, so that antibodies to HAV may be present as well. However, these will be of the IgG type, indicating an immune state.

Chronic Hepatitis B

Chronic hepatitis B develops when the immune reaction fails to obliterate the virus, resulting in a state of persistent low-grade inflammation of the liver. Cirrhosis is often already present when chronic hepatitis B is discovered. Serum ALT and AST are typically raised to levels of 100 to 500 U/dL (normal levels less than 70 and 50 U/dL, respectively) and occasionally higher. Bilirubin levels are often within normal limits. Surface antigen, core antibody (IgG type), and e antigen are present. Serum bilirubin levels are normal or only slightly elevated. Liver biopsy shows fibrosis or cirrhosis with variable degrees of inflammation. If the inflammation connects different areas of the liver within the biopsy, it is predictive of progression of the process. It is quite possible to be infected simultaneously with both HBV and HCV. In this case, antibody to hepatitis C will also be present.

It is important to be aware that, unlike in some other viral diseases (such as HIV, which causes AIDS) the load—that is, the number of virus particles present and measured by PCR—of HBV or HCV does not predict the outcome of the disease. The usefulness of PCR is to confirm the presence of the virus and determine response to treatment. Since successful treatment prevents replication of the virus, the number of viral particles as determined by the PCR is used to determine the response to therapy. A PCR is expensive and usually not necessary for diagnosis.

Management

Acute Hepatitis B
The treatment of acute hepatitis B is supportive; that is, there is no therapy that will shorten the course of the disease or lessen its severity. Nausea and vomiting can be treated, and dehydration can be prevented or treated with IV fluids. Hospitalization is to be avoided, although some 10 to 15 percent of those infected do require it. Since exercise does not influence liver function or tests, patients are encouraged to be up and about after the more bothersome symptoms subside. Additional rest does not speed recovery, and an early return to work is advised. Patients should be encouraged to do whatever they feel like doing. People with any form of hepatitis should be aware, however, that many with whom they come in contact will assume that the jaundice is infectious and transmissible. Drugs to control nausea and vomiting are often necessary and usually effective.

Chronic Hepatitis B

While no treatment cures cirrhosis, successful attacks on the virus slow or stop the chronic inflammation that leads to fibrosis and cirrhosis. Drugs that kill HBV or inhibit its growth and reproduction are interferon and lamivudine.

Interferon is one of the natural defense mechanisms against any virus. This compound has a direct antiviral effect as well as an immune-stimulating effect. While interferon can be isolated from the body in small amounts, it was not until the molecular structure was clarified and the compound could be produced in large amounts in the laboratory that it became available in sufficient quantities to allow use as treatment. There are several commercially available forms of interferon that differ slightly in structure. Clinical studies demonstrate no significant differences in their effectiveness against hepatitis viruses despite claims to the contrary.

Because interferon is a protein, it must be injected; stomach and intestinal secretions destroy it if taken by mouth. Furthermore, since it is foreign, the body's immune system reacts to it, with the first shot causing fever and chills. However, the body rapidly becomes tolerant of it, and, by the third shot, most patients do not have fever. Additional side effects include persistent malaise, depression that is usually mild but may be severe, sleep disturbances, temporary partial hair loss, and dysfunction of the thyroid, which may be either overactive or underactive. More potentially serious side effects include suppression of white blood cell and platelet production, resulting in reduction of the white cell and platelet counts, which makes the patient more susceptible to all infections and to bleeding. Expected and unexpected side effects should be carefully observed so that dosage can be decreased or the drug stopped if necessary. Interferon is seldom stopped altogether, but a reduction in dosage is sometimes required.

The immune system produces three different kinds of interferon, called interferon-alpha, interferon-beta, and interferon-gamma. The first of these, interferon α, was shown to be effective against both HBV and HCV. Interferon α has two effects on HBV. First, it seems to have a direct toxic effect on HBV (an "antiviral" effect), and, second, it directly stimulates the cellular immune system to more vigorously attack infected cells. For chronic hepatitis B, the usual dose of interferon is five million units daily for at least four and preferably six months. Some experts recommend ten million units three times each week for the same period. A slow-released form called pegylated interferon is now available in which only one injection per week is necessary. Those who have high ALT levels (reflecting active inflammation) and low numbers of HBV viral particles in their serum are more likely to respond. After an initial marked elevation of the ALT, about 60 percent of patients have reduction of their ALT to normal levels. Unfortunately, this response is not sustained in all infected persons. Only about 30 to 40 percent of those treated have no evidence of hepatitis as indicated by liver tests or biopsy and no HBV by PCR twelve months after treatment is ended. When interferon treatment is successful, surface antigen and e antigen are no longer present in serum, and antibody to both appears.

Treatment of chronic hepatitis B with interferon commonly results in an increase in serum ALT levels within the first four to six weeks of treatment. Levels of 1,000 to 2,000, compared to a normal of 40 U/dL, are not unusual. Jaundice may appear; fortunately, symptoms of acute hepatitis do not. Those who have such an initial elevation of ALT tend to respond more often with a sustained virological remission. The ALT is expected to decrease within three to four weeks while a person is still under treatment. Since an elevated ALT level reflects inflammation and death of liver cells, this initial response to interferon is also the reason that the drug cannot be used in cases of acute hepatitis or in those whose liver disease is so far advanced that they can ill afford even a minor and temporary decrease in function.

The second antiviral drug, lamivudine, is given in tablet form. Lamivudine prevents replication of the virus by interfering with enzymes essential to reproduction. Treatment with lamivudine in doses of 100 mg/day for six months is associated with normalization of liver tests in close to 100 percent of cases. Further, the viral counts by PCR fall to undetectable levels in most. When it is given for twelve months, at least half of patients show improvement in liver biopsy. The drug is well tolerated, with no symptoms or serious side effects. While this sounds wonderful, about 80 percent of patients have detectable virus again in six months after the drug is stopped. It has been suggested that lamivudine be used for long-term control of HBV in order to keep the inflammatory process suppressed, but no large studies published test this suggestion. Mutation of HBV that results in resistance to lamivudine sometimes occurs and would be a reason not to use this strategy. Studies are presently under way to test the effects of using interferon and lamivudine simultaneously. Preliminary indications are disappointing, but conclusions will depend on final results. Other antiviral drugs are being tested.

In those who develop severe symptomatic cirrhosis, liver transplantation affords good long-term survival rates. Although the new liver becomes infected with HBV and the resulting hepatitis can be severe, the course tends to be mild. Chronic disease typically progresses slowly but is suppressed by the drugs used against the immune system to prevent rejection of the transplanted liver.

Prevention

Obviously, avoiding behavior which puts a person at high risk for acquiring HBV is advisable. As noted, however, in a third of cases no such exposure has taken place (or is admitted to). For those who are known to have had recent exposure to a case of acute hepatitis, hyperimmune globulin against HBV, known as HBIG, is effective in preventing or ameliorating the disease. Hyperimmune globulin contains high levels of antibodies against HBV, having been collected from persons who are specifically selected because of their high levels of HBV antibodies.

Vaccines have been developed that are highly effective in inducing antibodies against HBsAg and, therefore, in preventing the disease. The cost is about $150 for the recommended series of three injections. In the United States, the vaccine is available in local health department clinics at a reduced cost.

Vaccines are made from purified surface antigen that is harvested from fungus in which the HBV surface antigen gene has been inserted. The vaccine contains only the surface antigen and no part of the virus. It cannot transmit the disease. It is given by injection in three doses over a period of six months and induces antibodies in about 90 percent of people. Since surface protein is essential for virus survival, antibodies destroy the virus before it becomes attached to the hepatic cell and causes infection. Those who are obese have a lower response rate than those of normal body weight, presumably because the vaccine is ineffectively absorbed from fatty tissue where it is injected. If those who do not develop antibodies undergo another series of injections, only about 10 percent will convert to an immune state. Interestingly, there is some evidence that those who receive the vaccine but do not develop antibodies are nevertheless partially protected when exposed.

The level of antibodies reaches a peak shortly after the second or third injection, and the antibodies persist for years with a slow reduction in measurable levels. By the tenth year, the levels are low or undetectable, and a booster shot every ten years is recommended by some. A normal trait of the immune system that has previously produced antibodies to an antigen is to retain the memory of how to do it—it does not have to relearn. Thus, reexposure to an antigen, such as that of HBV, results in an immediate outpouring of antibodies even when there are no measurable levels before exposure.

This is called the "anamnestic" response. Vaccination is recommended for all those adults at high risk for exposure, such as health care workers, those with multiple sexual partners (both male and female), and sexual partners of those known to be infected. Although the risk is small, it is ongoing for those living in the same house with someone who has chronic hepatitis B, and vaccination is recommended for them as well.

The American Academy of Pediatrics now strongly recommends that all children be vaccinated against hepatitis B, and the vaccine is being incorporated into the series of inoculations that children receive. Adolescents are also encouraged to receive the vaccine. Vaccines against both HAV and HBV can be effectively administered simultaneously.

In most obstetrical units, mothers are tested for HBV-surface antigen during pregnancy or when they come in for delivery. Newborns of mothers who test positive are inoculated immediately after delivery with hyperimmune globulin to provide immediate protection and are simultaneously given the first shot of vaccine for long-term protection, since they are at high risk for developing chronic hepatitis B.

5. Hepatitis C

Hepatitis C is serious not because it attacks the liver acutely but because it is seldom spontaneously eliminated. In fact, the acute disease, even when recognized, tends to be mild. Its persistence leads to cirrhosis in a significant number of those infected; it is a leading cause of that disease. Further, it predisposes to the development of hepatocellular carcinoma.

Prevalence

After hepatitis A and hepatitis B were identified, hepatitis still occurred following some blood transfusions, despite routinely applied tests for those diseases on donor blood. It had all the clinical characteristics of a hepatotrophic virus, and the disease was called non-A, non-B (NANB) hepatitis. It was responsible for over 85 percent of all cases of posttransfusion hepatitis before tests were developed to detect it. The virus was finally identified in 1989, and NANB was renamed hepatitis C virus (HCV). When blood tests for the virus became clinically available in about 1991, they began immediately to be applied to all donated blood, and the frequency of posttransfusion hepatitis fell dramatically. When large population groups were tested, HCV was found to be one of the most common chronic infections in the world.

The worldwide prevalence is estimated to be around 1 percent, with rates from 1 to 1.6 percent in North America and 10 to 14 percent in North Africa. An estimated 150–170 million people in the world are infected, compared to some 350 million with hepatitis B. Some 4 million people in the United States are presently harboring the virus, the great majority of whom are unaware of the infection. Fortunately, there is evidence that the rate of new infections has decreased by tenfold in the past ten years.

The majority of people who are infected do well. Our present treatment regimens, discussed below, are imperfect. We do not recommend treatment for everyone. Because of the large numbers of people involved, chronic hepatitis C is an important public health problem and should not be trivialized. Those who have it should be identified and offered treatment *if indicated*, but prognosis after infection is better than has been implied in the media. Most who are infected die with the disease but not because of it.

The Virus

HCV is an RNA virus (fig. 5.1) with nine major genotypes, designated by the numbers 1–9, of which only the first four (maybe five) are important players. There are at least forty different subtypes within these major types, designated by lowercase letters. The first genotype and subtype clearly identified was designated 1a. It is the most common genotype throughout the world and is associated with disease that is more severe than the others. Genotypes occur with varying frequency around the world and differ in their response to treatment. In the United States, genotype 1 is the most common, with subtype 1a being the most frequent subtype.

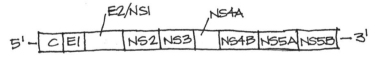

FIG. 5.1. Genome structure of the hepatitis C virus. The core (C) causes production of the basic or core protein of the virus. E1, E2, and NS1 cause production of the envelop proteins that coat each virus. NS2, NS3, NS4A, NS4B, NS5A, and NS5B are nonstructural proteins, which cause proteins to be produced that are not part of new viral particles but are important in replication.

Unfortunately, these two are the most resistant to treatment. Genotypes 2 and 3 are more common in Asia and make up about 10 percent and 6 percent, respectively, of the types in the United States. They are more responsive to treatment. Type 4 is common in the Near East, especially in Egypt, and is sometimes seen in the United States in people who have spent time in that part of the world. Types 5–9 are rare.

HCV readily mutates, resulting in closely related viruses called quasispecies within each major genotype. Several quasispecies may be present in the same individual. By virtue of natural selection, quasispecies tend to be more resistant to treatment than the parent virus and represent a mechanism by which the virus may escape host defenses and the effects of drugs. A quasispecies becomes predominant when less resistant forms are destroyed ("survival of the fittest"). We have a great deal more to learn about the significance of different species and quasispecies on prognosis and resistance to treatment.

HCV is destroyed by the acid environment of the stomach, so that fecal-oral transmission rarely occurs. The virus is transmitted by exchange of blood. As noted, all donated blood is tested, and transmission by this means is uncommon. The rate of hepatitis C is now less than one in one hundred thousand patients transfused and less than five for every ten thousand units of blood transfused.

The sharing of needles during "recreational" drug injection is the most common means of transmission. Many patients today are those who indulged in the "drug culture" of the 1960s (if only for a little while—once is enough). This should in no way be taken to mean that infection with HCV proves that the individual used IV drugs in the past. As with hepatitis B, around 20 to 40 percent of infected persons have no identifiable risk factors. Educational efforts and the appearance of AIDS have resulted in less sharing of needles and therefore a decrease in the number of new cases of hepatitis C. Health care personnel can become infected despite careful protective measures. Transmission may also occur through kidney dialysis units where considerable amounts of blood are used. In such units, the prevalence of antibodies has been reported to be between 10 and 20 percent compared to 1.5 percent in a similar population not being dialyzed.

Transmission by sexual intercourse or to members of a household, while known to occur, is unusual. In monogamous relationships involving one partner who is infected but whose liver tests are normal, the sexual partner is found to be infected in less than 3 percent of cases. Even when the infected spouse has active disease with abnormal liver tests, less than 7 percent of the uninfected spouses acquire the disease if they do not have other risk factors. The incidence of HCV in male and female prostitutes and homosexuals is only slightly higher than in the general population.

Transmission from mothers with the virus to their newborn infants occurs infrequently. It should be noted that, at birth, infants of mothers who have HCV antibodies will also have maternal antibodies that have crossed the placenta but no evidence that the virus is present. These maternal antibodies in the infant will disappear after several months. If the mother is infected with HIV in addition to HCV, a not-uncommon occurrence, the risk to the child of being infected at birth with HCV is markedly increased.

The Disease

Acute Hepatitis C

Acute hepatitis C is rarely recognized because its symptoms are usually mild and go unnoticed. Because of this, it is difficult to confidently estimate the total number of infections and the number of people who manage to eliminate the virus. From those cases that have been seen in the acute phase, it appears that not more than 15 percent are able to overcome the virus completely. It should be noted, however, that the eventual outcome of chronic HCV infection is actually good in the majority of patients. In one large study, almost six hundred people who developed posttransfusion hepatitis, 72 percent of whom were later proven to have the virus, were compared to over nine hundred people who had also received transfusions but did not get hepatitis. After an average of eighteen years the number of all deaths due to any cause was the same in both groups, although there were more deaths associated with liver disease (3.3 percent) in those who had hepatitis than in those who did not (1.5 percent). There was no difference in death rates between those who had hepatitis C and those who did not.

Jaundice is usually not present. The ALT level is often never more than 250 U/dL in the acute phase and may be higher in the chronic phase. Nausea and vomiting are uncommon.

As in all forms of viral hepatitis, HCV does not seem to directly destroy hepatic cells. Elimination is accomplished by destruction of infected liver cells by the cellular immune system. The immune response to HCV is characteristically less than vigorous. This appears to be why only a minority of those infected rid themselves of the virus, and chronic hepatitis is the rule rather than the exception. The relatively weak immune response probably also accounts for the rarity of acute liver failure in HCV.

Chronic Hepatitis C

Chronic hepatitis C, as defined by the liver biopsy, develops in the majority of patients who become infected. Most of those have no symptoms. In people who do, the most common is chronic fatigue that is disproportionate to the amount of disease in the liver. Depression seems to be more frequent than in other diseases. Other symptoms are equally nonspecific and include loss of appetite, nausea with little or no vomiting, vague abdominal discomfort localized over the liver, and joint pains with no swelling.

At least 85 percent of those infected with HCV have hepatitis on liver biopsy, but severity is variable. In the majority of people, it is mild or moderate. Serial liver biopsies show that inflammation is persistent over years and tends to cause progressive fibrosis with variable rapidity. Liver tests may be consistently normal and, in these, the majority have minimal changes or even a normal liver biopsy. Once established, the virus rarely disappears spontaneously. The major risk of chronic hepatitis is progressive fibrosis which, when fully developed, is cirrhosis. In long-term observations about 20 percent of patients with chronic hepatitis C develop cirrhosis after an average of twenty years. According to two studies published in 1999, the frequency may be only 5 to 10 percent. In one study, 62,667 women were identified as having received a globulin preparation later found to be possibly contaminated with HCV. All were traced. Seven hundred and four had evidence of past or current HCV infection and 390 (55 percent) had a PCR showing HCV RNA. Seventeen years later, 390 (1.1 percent) showed evidence of HCV and 376 agreed to be evaluated. About half of these had elevated levels of AST, but only 8 percent had levels over a hundred. The majority had symptoms, chiefly fatigue. Only seven (2 percent) were found to have cirrhosis, although 98 percent had at least mild hepatitis on liver biopsy. In another study, seventeen servicemen were examined after their blood, frozen forty-five years before, was found to be infected. Of these seventeen, two (12 percent) were found to have cirrhosis.

Although the public perception is that cirrhosis of the liver is usually caused by alcohol abuse, it is more often the result of some other problem, such as chronic hepatitis C. It is also commonly assumed that anyone who has cirrhosis will eventually die from it. It can indeed be life threatening, but in about half of those with chronic hepatitis C found to have cirrhosis by biopsy, there are no signs or symptoms of that disease. Therefore, if cirrhosis occurs in 20 percent or less of people with chronic hepatitis C and only half of those have any signs of that disease, it follows that less than 10 percent are at risk for death from liver disease. Nevertheless, because such a large number of people are infected with HCV, it is the most common cause of cirrhosis in the United States.

The combination of even moderate amounts of alcohol and HCV leads to cirrhosis at a rate that is at least tenfold greater than if alcohol is not consumed. Furthermore, in those who have a drinking problem, 15 percent to as many as 60 percent have chronic hepatitis C. The reason for this synergistic effect between alcohol and HCV is unknown. Obviously, those with chronic hepatitis C are well advised to abstain from alcohol.

HCV may cause other disorders not directly involving the liver. Occurring in a minority of infected people, these are referred to as extrahepatic manifestations and include a type of serious inflammatory kidney disease called glomerulonephritis that causes loss of protein in the urine, reduction in renal function, and hypertension. Inflammation of blood vessels (vasculitis) has been observed, as has fibrosis of the lungs and rheumatoid arthritis. Rheumatoid factor, an antibody found in the blood of rheumatoid arthritis patients, is often present in chronic hepatitis C. HCV predisposes to the formation of an abnormal circulating protein called cryoglobulin. This peculiar protein precipitates out of blood when the temperature falls below normal body temperature, as commonly occurs in the digits and limbs. Capillaries may be obstructed by these precipitates, leading to skin rashes and tiny hemorrhages. Generally, however, cryoglobulinemia associated with HCV causes no signs or symptoms. A metabolic disease associated with destructive sun sensitivity of the skin and an intermittent red urine called porphyria cutanea tarda may also occur.

Chronic hepatitis C is also associated with abnormal accumulation of iron in the liver, probably due to a shortened life of red blood cells, which contain large amounts of iron.

When these cells are destroyed, the released iron is taken up by the liver. Excess iron in the liver has been associated with a poor response to treatment, and improvement in response to treatment when iron is removed by periodic bloodletting has been both claimed and denied. Because of the disorders associated with HCV, a search for the virus when one of these is present is advisable, with the hope that treatment will decrease their frequency or severity.

In those with cirrhosis, the frequency of hepatocellular carcinoma (HCC) is markedly increased. It is estimated that about 5 percent of these will develop HCC, representing a relative risk that is increased some 250 times in these patients compared to the U.S. population in general. Cirrhosis of any cause is associated with HCC but to a lesser degree than that associated with HCV or HBV.

Diagnosis

Acute Hepatitis C

The signs, symptoms, and laboratory findings of acute hepatitis C are indistinguishable from those of any of the hepatotrophic virus and have been described in chapter 2. Acute cases are seldom seen for reasons already noted, but hepatitis C must be considered in the differential diagnosis of any case of acute hepatitis. Because antibodies against HCV do not appear until about eight to ten weeks after onset of the disease, tests for them are not useful in recently acquired disease. However, the virus appears in the serum early on and can be quantified by amplification of HCV RNA using the PCR. The PCR is therefore useful for identifying the acute disease. Liver biopsy that shows hepatitis will not define its cause and thus is not helpful. When these tools are used, the diagnosis of acute hepatitis due to HCV is seldom a problem.

Chronic Hepatitis C

Chronic hepatitis C is usually discovered when laboratory tests are done for any reason and abnormal liver tests are found. In most cases, the physical examination is completely normal, but in some, the liver may be moderately enlarged and slightly tender. If extensive fibrosis or cirrhosis is present, the liver and spleen are enlarged and palpable. Signs of cirrhosis (see chapter 2) include fluid in the abdomen (ascites), swelling (edema) of the legs, and hepatic "spiders."

Antibodies to HCV (see table 5.1) are detected by the ELISA, or enzyme-linked immunosorbent assay, which tests for two antigens (called C_{100}/C_{33} fusion protein and C_{22}, a core protein), the sensitivity and specificity of which is about 98 percent and 95 percent, respectively. That is, in those people with risk factors such as the receiving of blood transfusions before we could test for the disease or IV drug abuse, ELISA will detect antibodies to the virus when present about 98 percent of the time (it will miss 2 percent of cases) and will be negative when the virus is not present 95 percent of the time (it will be falsely positive in 5 percent of those without antibodies to the virus). In those with no identifiable risk factors, the sensitivity and specificity is about 85 percent and 80 percent, respectively. These antibodies do not reflect immunity (are not protective against the disease) but indicate that the virus is or has been present. Once present, anti-HCV antibodies remain detectable for the life of the individual *even if treatment is successful in obliterating the virus.*

A second test is the RIBA, or radioimmunoblot assay, for antigens of the virus genome. It can be used in those regarding whom there is some doubt about the validity of the ELISA test, but it is now seldom employed because the more sensitive PCR test for the RNA of HCV is readily available.

The presence of virus can be documented by a qualitative PCR, which detects the presence of the RNA of the virus and costs about $150. The quantitative test measures the number of viral RNA particles and is much more expensive ($250-$600). The number of viral RNA particles must be high enough to be detected. Levels as low as one hundred viruses per ml of blood can be detected. If the number of RNA particles is below the sensitivity of the method, the result is reported as "below detectable," since virus could be present in low numbers. A qualitative PCR is helpful when liver tests are normal but the ELISA test is positive. In such a case, the absence of virus by PCR is evidence that the ELISA test is falsely positive. Although it is possible to have the virus and a positive antibody test but a negative PCR, this circumstance is often due to the mishandling of one of the blood specimens.

In a national conference held in 1997 and sponsored by the National Institutes of Health, a panel of experts concluded that a liver biopsy should be done in all cases and treatment based on the findings. Since then, experience suggests that a liver biopsy is not routinely necessary, especially when the decision to treat has already been made. As pointed out elsewhere, liver tests only generally reflect the status of the liver, and a biopsy is helpful in determining the stage of the disease, the degree of inflammation, and whether or not cirrhosis is already present. In the presence of the virus and completely normal liver tests, it may still be argued that liver biopsy will show severe hepatitis in a few and that these cases should be treated. No consensus has developed on this question. The official recommendation by the National Institutes of Health is that people with the virus but repeatedly normal liver tests or less than one and a half times the upper limits of normal (over at least three months) do not obtain sufficient benefit to justify the treatment risks, discomforts, and costs, and should not be treated.

Management

Treatment for hepatitis C is a combination of interferon α and ribavirin. (See chapter 4 for a description of interferon α and its side effects.) Whether we should treat the disease when it is recognized in its acute phase is arguable. Most of us with experience will do so in the appropriate setting. The hesitancy comes from knowing that in acute hepatitis B, interferon α cannot be used because it temporarily makes that disease worse. This does not occur in hepatitis C, and, because the majority with acute hepatitis C develop persistent infection and chronic liver disease, use of interferon α seems rational. There have been only a few studies in a relatively small number of patients regarding this issue, but the findings suggest a much higher rate of complete disease remission (39 to 40 percent) in those with acute hepatitis C treated with IFN at an early stage compared with untreated subjects (0 percent). On the other hand, treatment of the patient with severe cirrhosis and very abnormal liver tests with jaundice (called "decompensated") should not receive treatment because of the risk of making the inflammatory process temporarily worse and causing the death of the patient.

Treatment is recommended for those with liver enzymes (ALT and AST) that are persistently more than one and a half times the upper limit of normal. One of the peculiar characteristics of chronic hepatitis C is that liver tests have a tendency to fluctuate widely from normal to markedly abnormal at variable intervals, usually within weeks. Therefore, if a normal ALT is found, it must be repeated over a period of time, usually three months, before the conclusion may be reached that liver tests are persistently normal. To determine that treatment is not indicated, *persistently* normal ALT levels must be documented. Of those with inactive disease, a few may later have active disease without symptoms or signs. Thus, it is advisable for them to have liver tests every six to twelve months indefinitely.

The aim of treatment is to rid the body of virus; when this is accomplished, it is referred to as a virologic response to treatment. Before treatment is started, a quantitative PCR to measure the number of viral RNA particles present (the viral load) is done. While the viral load in some viral diseases directly predicts the eventual outcome, this is not true in chronic hepatitis C. Its use is in determining the viral response to treatment. If the viral load does not fall at least tenfold after twelve to sixteen weeks, the prediction can be made that treatment will fail and it can be stopped, there being no need for the usual forty-eight weeks.

It is cost effective to determine the genotype. Genotypes 2 and 3 are more likely than genotype 1 to be obliterated with only twenty-four weeks of treatment. Longer treatment for genotypes 2 and 3 does not improve treatment response rates.

Interferon α is self-administered as injections of 3 million units three times a week for forty-eight weeks in genotype 1 (both 1a and 1b) and for twenty-four weeks in genotypes 2 and 3. Some patients are more tolerant of the drug if it is given every other night. There is a marginal increase in the initial response if interferon is administered daily in a dose of 5 million units for thirty days followed by 3 million units three times a week thereafter. This is called induction therapy. When interferon is given alone (monotherapy) the response of abnormal liver tests, chiefly the ALT, is about 50 percent. Unfortunately, relapse occurs in most of these within three to six months. The aim, however, is a virologic response as determined by levels of virus below detectable limits by PCR, and this occurs in only about 15 percent of those treated with monotherapy. Therefore, interferon is combined with ribavirin to increase the virologic response. Long-term virologic response when this combination is used is approximately 40 percent. In those who cannot take ribavirin for whatever reason, monotherapy is recommended. Long-term studies comparing patients who refused treatment with interferon monotherapy to those who were treated but did not respond show that treated patients fare better than untreated ones, with a lower frequency of cirrhosis and of hepatocellular carcinoma years later. Combination therapy has not been in use long enough to do such studies, but one can assume similar results.

For reasons not understood, African Americans respond very poorly to both interferon monotherapy and combination therapy with interferon and ribavirin. Ribavirin has no effect on HCV when used alone. It does not change the side effects of interferon α. Ribavirin is generally well tolerated. Cough and shortness of breath have been reported in a minority of those using it. Ribavirin routinely causes some destruction of older red blood cells. A fall in hemoglobin of about three grams in the first three weeks of treatment is expected, and a few will have an even greater fall. The levels become stable at the lowered level where they persist throughout treatment. Frequent blood counts are necessary to insure that hemoglobin levels do not become dangerously low (anemia). Such a rapid fall in hemoglobin puts the patient with ischemic heart disease (often identified by angina or an abnormal EKG) at risk of a myocardial infarction (heart attack). These patients should be treated with caution or excluded from ribavirin treatment. Similarly, patients with renal insufficiency are excluded, because the kidneys do not have enough reserve function to handle the increased load of bilirubin with which they are they presented when ribavirin causes a sudden rapid destruction of red blood cells.

Hemoglobin before treatment must be above 12 grams% in all. If the level falls below 10.5 grams%, the dose of ribavirin is halved, and if below 8.5 grams%, ribavirin must be stopped. A complete blood count (CBC) must be done two weeks after initiation of ribavirin and once each month for the duration of treatment. Occasionally patients develop an allergy to ribavirin, indicated by a rash, in which case it should be stopped immediately.

In experimental animals, ribavirin administered to either males or females induces a high rate of spontaneous abortion or of fetal abnormalities in the progeny. This effect seems to persist for as long as six months following use. Thus, it is to be used with caution in people of reproductive age and only with effective contraception. Routine pregnancy tests are recommended during use and for six months afterward.

During treatment, liver tests are obtained on a regular basis at the discretion of the physician. Occasionally, autoimmune liver disease (see chapter 6) will also be present despite efforts to detect it before treatment is initiated. It may, in fact, be induced by HCV. Interferon α has an adverse effect on this disease, causing striking elevations of ALT levels, and interferon must be discontinued.

Patients who have a virologic response at the end of treatment have a 90 percent chance of being virus free indefinitely. If viral RNA levels by PCR are still below detectable levels six months after the last treatment, there is approximately a 95 percent chance of absence of virus indefinitely. In order to detect those few in whom the virus reappears, liver tests and a qualitative PCR should be obtained twelve months after completion of treatment; that will determine who has relapsed (i.e., who has not had a sustained response). A small number will relapse later. For this reason, annual liver tests and qualitative PCR are advisable for at least two additional years.

Patients who remain in remission do not progress to cirrhosis. Further, a few studies suggest that there is a decrease in the amount of fibrosis in those who remain in remission for three to five years. The risk of hepatocellular carcinoma is considerably diminished but not entirely absent.

In 1999 several cases of acute hepatitis A were reported in patients with chronic hepatitis C. These patients did not do well, and some deaths occurred as a result of acute liver failure. Based on these few cases, it is recommended that all patients with chronic hepatitis C be vaccinated against hepatitis A. The vaccine is safe and effective in such circumstances. Many physicians will also recommend vaccination against hepatitis B.

The cost of forty-eight weeks of treatment with interferon and ribavirin, including periodic laboratory studies, is approximately four thousand to six thousand dollars. The pharmaceutical companies that make interferon have programs in place to assist those who need it with these costs (see appendix for addresses).

Prevention

The incidence of hepatitis C is falling. This is partly because of testing for the presence of the virus in donor blood and in biological agents that are made from blood and injected for various treatments, such as concentrated factor VII for bleeding disorders. Unfortunately, vaccines are not available. Efforts to develop them continue, but the results are not encouraging. Although the use of gamma globulin has not been specifically tested as prophylaxis against HCV, studies with this preparation several years ago in efforts to prevent posttransfusion hepatitis, which was primarily caused by HCV, were unsuccessful. Since there is no reason to believe that gamma globulin would be helpful, it is not recommended. Tattoos and body piercing have been implicated and should be avoided. The sharing of needles during illicit drug use is now the most common mode of transmission.

Table 5.1. Antibody Tests for Hepatitis A, B, and C

Agent	Term	Definition	Significance
Hepatitis A virus (**HAV**)	Anti-HAV	Antibody against HAV:	
	IgG	Present after acute infection	Present for years; immunity
	IgM	During acute infection	Acute infection is present
Hepatitis B virus (**HBV**)	HBsAg	Surface antigen (Ag) of virus	Present in acute, chronic, or carrier stages
	Anti-HBsAg (surface antibody)	Antibody to surface antigen	Immune state
	HBcAb (core antibody)	Antibody to core antigen	
	IgG	After acute infection	Past infection
	IgM	During acute activity	Active hepatitis B
	HBeAg	e antigen of virus	Viral replication
	Anti-HBe	e antibody	No viral replication
Hepatitis C virus (**HCV**)	Anti-HCV	Antibody to C virus	8–16 weeks after infection Not protective; virus present in 95%+

Table 5.2. Characteristics of Hepatitis A, B, and C

Cause	A (HAV) RNA virus	B (HBV) DNA virus	C (HCV) RNA virus
Transmission	Fecal-oral Food and water	Blood exchange Intimate contact	Blood exchange
Incubation period	2–6 weeks	4–16 weeks	5–10 weeks
Period of infectivity	Late incubation and for 2 weeks after jaundice	During HBsAg positive period	During HCV positive period
Acute liver failure	Rare	Uncommon	Rare
Carrier state	No	Yes	Yes
Chronic hepatitis	No	Yes	Yes
Vaccine	Yes	Yes	No

HAV=hepatitis A virus; HBV=hepatitis B virus; HCV=hepatitis C virus; HBsAg=hepatitis B surface antigen indicating that the virus is present; carrier state=a person with no clinical signs of liver disease (normal liver tests) but who has HBsAg in his or her serum

6. Other Viruses and Nonviral Causes of Hepatitis

Other Viral Causes of Hepatitis

Hepatitis D virus (fig. 6.1) occurs rarely in the United States, but is common in the Amazon basin, parts of Africa, and around the Mediterranean. It is sometimes seen here in visitors from those areas. HDV is defective and requires the presence of HBV (its "helper virus") to reproduce. If hepatitis B virus is not present, neither is the hepatitis D virus. Acute hepatitis D may occur in those who have chronic hepatitis B, or the two viruses may infect simultaneously. The acute clinical picture of hepatitis D is indistinguishable from that of hepatitis A, B, or C and commonly causes chronic hepatitis. Acute hepatitis D is suspected when a patient with known chronic hepatitis B suddenly develops another episode

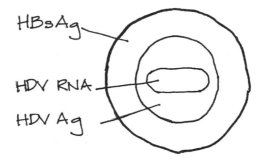

FIG. 6.1. Hepatitis D virus. Note that, like HAV, the genome is only a single RNA structure.

of acute hepatitis. While this can be the result of an exacerbation of hepatitis B, a superinfection with hepatitis D would be considered in those areas in which HDV is known to occur. Both chronic disease and acute liver failure occur with acute hepatitis D with a higher frequency than with other hepatotrophic viruses. The presence of antibodies against HDV is diagnostic.

The hepatitis E virus (HEV) was first recognized in India and is transmitted by the fecal-oral route, just as is HAV. HEV has not occurred in the United States so far, but it has been seen in sporadic cases in people who have traveled here from India. This virus is a potential threat to the U.S. population since it has been identified in North America in one small epidemic in Mexico. The virus is highly infectious and unique in that infected pregnant women, as well as their fetuses, have a high mortality rate. Women who are not pregnant and men seldom die of the disease. To date, no cases of chronic hepatitis E have been found.

There is no hepatitis virus "F" because that designation was assigned to a misidentified organism that was found not to be a hepatotrophic virus.

Hepatitis G virus (HGV) is a common virus that, although hepatotrophic, has not been shown to cause any significant changes in the liver, either acute or chronic. It can be identified in a large portion of people who have received blood transfusions or have been exposed to substances made from blood, such as plasma. We do not test for this inconsequential virus.

Transfusion transmitted virus (TTV) was first identified in Japan and subsequently in other countries including the United States. Like HGV, it seems to cause little damage to the liver or any other organ and is not considered an important infectious agent.

Cases of acute hepatitis occur that closely resemble hepatitis caused by the known viruses, but are not. Their clinical presentation is indistinguishable from other forms of viral hepatitis, but antibodies against known hepatotrophic viruses are not present. The prevalence of non-A-E disease (or diseases—there may be more than one) is unknown, but virtually every physician who sees patients with hepatitis has seen at least one or more. This putative hepatotrophic virus has not been isolated or identified, but studies are under way to do so. Perhaps it will eventually be renamed hepatitis I (or F?).

We know virtually nothing about the non-A-E agent(s) except that it acts like a hepatotrophic virus. Indeed, if all cases of acute liver failure are examined, 30 to 40 percent have no identifiable agent. The "unknown virus(s)" may be responsible for a significant number of these. It has been associated with suppression of bone marrow function, resulting in sometimes critically low levels of the cells produced by this organ—decreases in red blood cells can cause anemia, in platelets can lead to spontaneous bleeding, and in white blood cells can make the patient susceptible to overwhelming bacterial infection. We do not know if non-A-E can cause chronic hepatitis, and no antibody has been identified to date. We have much to learn.

Many viruses that are not primarily hepatotrophic may cause hepatitis. Fortunately, the vast majority have been unknown in the United States during the last century. The most notorious of these are the hemorrhagic viruses, which include yellow fever, Lassa fever, Marburg, ebola, Rift Valley fever virus, and others. These forms of hepatitis are often the subjects of news reports about epidemics with high case fatality rates in areas of the world far removed from the United States.

The hemorrhagic viruses cause general destruction of red blood cells, interference with normal clotting of blood, and marked damage to small blood vessels. There is jaundice of variable intensity, massive hemorrhage into the gastrointestinal tract, and kidney failure. Case fatality rates vary from 10 percent to over 90 percent. Each of these viruses is transmitted between humans and animals by mosquito bites. The organs primarily damaged vary, but hepatitis is common in all and is routinely present in yellow fever.

Yellow fever, once common in the southern United States, is now of only historical interest. Dr. Walter Reed, for whom the military hospital in Washington, D.C., was named, identified the vector (the *Aedes aegypti* mosquito). The last case in the Americas was in Trinidad in 1954.

Yellow fever is now uncommon in most of the world, but there are pockets in Africa and South America where a recent surge of cases has occurred. In the five years from 1987 to 1991, there were 18,735 cases, with 4,522 deaths reported to the World Health Organization (WHO), the greatest five-year number since 1948. An effective vaccine is available. Mosquitoes transmit the disease between animals (chiefly monkeys) and humans. The organism replicates in both liver and muscle cells and apparently directly causes cell death. The disease is commonly associated with kidney failure resulting from damage to the small vessels essential to normal kidney function.

The cause of dengue fever is also a hemorrhagic virus, although the disease is generally less severe than those discussed above. In most cases, generally mild hepatitis occurs. It is a potential threat for epidemics in the United States. In 1999, there was one death in over fifty cases of dengue fever in Texas.

Infectious mononucleosis (the "kissing disease") is caused by Epstein-Barr virus, which is transmitted by saliva. This disease is marked by generalized swelling of lymph nodes, spleen, and inflammation of the throat. It can last for several weeks and is often followed by several months of chronic fatigue and ill health. An elevated white count, anemia, and low platelet counts may persist for several months, although laboratory abnormalities are usually normal within four to twelve weeks. In blood, lymphocytes outnumber other white blood cells, in contrast to the normal circumstance. Epstein-

Barr virus causes the appearance of antibodies that do not attack the virus but cause clumping and disruption of ox or horse red blood cells. This is called "heterophile" antibody and is routinely used to make a diagnosis. The characteristic pattern of liver tests in this disease is moderate elevation of the ALT and AST and a marked elevation of serum alkaline phosphatase levels. This pattern contrasts sharply with liver tests in hepatitis A, B, and C and can be confusing. This form of hepatitis can be severe enough to cause death from liver failure, although the frequency is uncertain. The Epstein-Barr virus is also implicated in certain forms of malignancy of lymph nodes (lymphoma) unrelated to hepatitis.

A particularly virulent form of hepatitis is caused by herpes simplex virus (HSV). Two closely related forms of this virus are called HSV-1 and HSV-2. HSV-2 is strongly associated with skin and genital infections, whereas HSV-1 can infect other organs, including the liver. Inflammation of the brain (encephalitis) caused by HSV-1 leads to death in almost 30 percent of cases. HSV-1 hepatitis is generally devastating, causing virtually complete destruction of liver, and has a high mortality rate. This form of hepatitis is rare and is generally restricted to people whose immune system is severely compromised, such as those who have any severe or prolonged illness, including AIDS, or who have had an organ transplant. A diagnosis can be made by direct culture of the virus on special media.

Cytomegalovirus is, as the name implies, an unusually large one; it circulates continuously in our population, seldom causing disease. Most adults have antibodies in their serum, indicating a previous exposure. Hepatitis caused by cytomegalovirus is infrequent and usually mild. It is transmitted largely by children but can also follow sexual contact. It does not lead to epidemics. Although it seldom causes hepatitis, it can do so in patients whose immune system is depressed by illness or drugs. Cytomegalovirus disease is common in patients who have had liver or other organ transplants because of the immune-suppressing drugs necessary to prevent rejection.

Certain childhood viral diseases may be complicated by hepatitis on rare occasions. These include mumps, measles (rubeola), "German" or "three-day" measles (rubella), and chicken pox (varicella). In children, these forms of hepatitis are generally confined to abnormal liver tests, including mild jaundice, and rapidly resolve, but can be severe if they occur in adults. Vaccines now used routinely in children have markedly reduced the frequency of these childhood diseases and thus their complications.

Alcoholic Hepatitis

Only humans drink alcohol voluntarily. Animals do so only when given no choice. Alcohol in large amounts is toxic to the liver. This effect is not prevented by an adequate food intake. These two facts were best documented in a small number of healthy volunteers who drank a measured amount (about a fifth—750 ml) of 80 proof (40 percent) alcohol daily for about five days while consuming a nutritious diet. Liver biopsies were done before and after the experimental period and demonstrated a distinct change from no fat to significant fat accumulation in all subjects. Fortunately, these abnormalities are reversible if alcohol is withdrawn early. Fat accumulation is the first, but reversible, step in the development of alcoholic hepatitis. If a group of chronic alcoholics are examined by liver biopsy, about one-fourth will have normal livers, one-third will have fatty liver only, one-fifth will have acute inflammation (alcoholic hepatitis) without cirrhosis, and one-fourth will have cirrhosis.

Alcoholic hepatitis is dependant on (1) average daily consumption, (2) duration of the abuse, and to some unknown degree on genetic predisposition. Women are more susceptible, for example, to alcoholic liver injury than men. Currently accepted data suggest that daily intake of eighty grams of alcohol per day in men and forty grams per day in women for five years will result in permanent liver injury. Because of variation in the response of individuals, limits of sixty grams for men and twenty grams for women have been recommended.

One ounce of 80 proof whiskey (40 percent alcohol) contains approximately ten grams of alcohol. Therefore a half pint of whiskey contains eighty grams. A six-pack of twelve-ounce cans of beer (3.5 percent) contains about seventy-six grams, while seven hundred fifty ml of wine (12.5 percent) contains about seventy-two grams. Daily intake of these amounts for over five years engenders the risk of irreversible liver damage. Intake greater than eighty to one hundred grams per day over a shorter period will regularly result in acute hepatitis, but it is generally reversible when alcohol is withdrawn. Contrary to common belief, it is alcohol that is injurious, and the form in which it is consumed is of no consequence. Switching from liquor to beer does not protect the liver.

Liver changes in alcoholics occur as follows (the intermediate stage of alcoholic hepatitis may be bypassed):

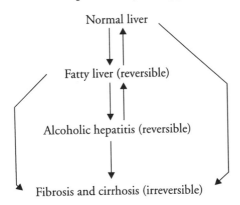

Normal liver

Fatty liver (reversible)

Alcoholic hepatitis (reversible)

Fibrosis and cirrhosis (irreversible)

Patients with alcoholic liver disease are commonly malnourished, but it has not been explicitly proven that concurrent malnutrition and alcoholism are additive. On the other hand, malnutrition has been repeatedly shown to increase morbidity and mortality in a host of diseases, and alcoholic liver disease is not an exception. One can assume that it is better to have one disease at a time!

Alcohol injures the liver by several mechanisms. It causes accumulation of fat by interfering with its release. Fatty liver is the first change that can be seen with the light microscope, but the condition is rapidly reversed when alcohol is no longer present. Such an accumulation causes enlargement of the whole organ and may be so severe that individual fat cells rupture, forming fatty cysts. Release of fat into tissue between cells causes an inflammatory reaction, that, if persistent, leads to fibrosis and eventually to cirrhosis.

Alcohol interferes with multiple metabolic functions and increases the demand for oxygen within each hepatic cell. It is metabolized to a compound called acetaldehyde that can join with proteins to form antigens. Cells that are in the process of being destroyed by alcohol form accumulations of residual intracellular elements called tubulin. Tubulin is the material that forms an internal skeleton of all cells and helps them maintain their shape. This accumulated material stains red with the dyes used to make the cells more visible under the microscope and is called Mallory bodies. While Mallory bodies are characteristic of alcoholic liver disease, they can be seen with other forms of injury and are thus not specific to alcohol injury. For example, they are regularly seen in nonalcoholic steatohepatitis, or NASH syndrome (discussed later in this chapter). They are no longer referred to by their old name, which was Mallory's alcoholic hyaline.

Inflammation stimulates stellate cells, normal cells of the liver, to change their form and their function. Stellate cells normally store vitamin A, but, under these conditions, begin to secrete a substance called collagen, the protein of fibrous tissue. If the injury continues, fibrosis becomes more and more dense until, finally, cirrhosis is present. Fibrosis or even cirrhosis is already present in 25 percent or more of those found to have alcoholic hepatitis for the first time.

As usual, liver tests are not diagnostic. If jaundice is present, the serum bilirubin is necessarily elevated. Since fatty liver is common and because fat in the liver partially obstructs small bile ducts, the serum alkaline phosphatase is usually elevated. Although serum ALT is characteristically elevated more than serum AST in most forms of hepatitis, the reverse is true in alcoholic hepatitis. If the AST/ALT ratio is greater than two to one, alcoholic hepatitis is probable. The unusually low ALT may be due to a deficiency of pyridoxine (vitamin B_6). As nutrition improves and pyridoxine is ingested, the ALT level commonly rises above normal before it falls back into the normal range.

Acute alcoholic hepatitis resolves in time in 90 percent of patients when alcohol is withdrawn. Liver tests become normal in about six to twelve weeks, but liver biopsy shows that the acute process may take six to twelve months to completely resolve. In about 10 percent of cases, the injury continues despite absence of alcohol intake. Immunity may play some role in this persistent disease. For example, antibodies against Mallory bodies can be demonstrated in a high portion of those with alcoholic hepatitis. Furthermore, antibodies against an antigen made up of a combination of acetaldehyde, the principle metabolite of alcohol, and proteins have been found in some patients. At this time, it is still uncertain why a minority of those with acute alcoholic hepatitis do not recover from it.

Severe alcoholic hepatitis is marked by intense jaundice with serum bilirubin levels above 5–10 mg/dL. Patients who have it are sometimes given steroids in the form of prednisone or prednisolone (known suppressants of the inflammatory process), orally or intravenously, to speed recovery, although the effectiveness of this is open to question. Those with less severe disease do not benefit from steroid therapy.

A problem with interpreting what we thought we knew about alcoholic liver disease is presented by the relatively recent identification of hepatitis C (see chapter 5). As pointed out previously, the frequency of chronic hepatitis C in patients with alcoholic liver disease is at least ten times and in some populations forty times the frequency in nonalcoholics. Further, alcoholics who are infected with hepatitis C are known to have a faster progression of their viral disease and a greater frequency of cirrhosis than those who do not drink alcohol. What this means is that a great deal of data we have on liver disease in alcoholics may have been related in whole or in part to the unsuspected presence of HCV. Data need to be re-collected with added tests for HCV.

Hepatitis Caused by Drugs

Many compounds, both those occurring naturally and those manufactured for medicinal use, can cause injury to organs. Common over-the-counter (OTC) or nonprescription drugs such as acetaminophen (Tylenol), aspirin, laxatives, cough syrups, and others are safe in recommended doses, but greater amounts can be hepatotoxic. Similarly, liver injury due to prescription drugs is remarkably infrequent, about one to five per million people who take them. A few drugs, notably some used to treat tuberculosis or epilepsy, have rates of about one to two per hundred but continue to be used, albeit with caution, because they are highly effective and no substitutes are available.

Low rates of adverse reactions are due to exhaustive investigations that each drug undergoes before it is released for medicinal use. Before approval for marketing by the U.S. Food and Drug Administration (FDA), a new drug must be proven both safe and effective. Unregulated treatments, on the other hand, such as herbs, may contain potentially damaging chemicals, and few have been investigated for safety and efficacy.

Drug-induced hepatitis may be caused by the drug itself or by its breakdown products. The many mechanisms by which such injury occurs are complex and will not be covered here. Allergic reactions to drugs are well known, but the liver is usually only peripherally involved in such reactions. Immune reactions can occur when the drug or one of its breakdown products combines with a protein of the body to form an antigen. Some adverse reactions are a combination of chemical and immunologic injury. A third kind of reaction, called idiosyncratic, is rare and due to an unexpected and therefore unpredictable hypersensitivity that is unique to an individual. In addition, some drugs will interfere with the actions of other drugs, resulting in loss of efficacy, failure to metabolize (leading to an accumulation of a drug to toxic levels), or other cross-reactions that are harmful.

A list of every drug that has been reported to cause chemical hepatitis at least once would be a long one. Some are known to cause some degree of hepatitis more often than others. Liver tests are periodically performed when these are used. Suffice it to say that physicians consider all drugs as potential causes of hepatitis. Only a few will be mentioned here.

Drug hepatitis can show itself in several ways. The more subtle presentation is by abnormal liver tests when there are no signs or symptoms. Because some drugs are known to cause such a reaction, liver tests are routinely checked when they are prescribed. One example is some of the antituberculosis drugs, especially one called isoniazid (there are several brand names). Because of chronic inflammation with resultant fibrosis, failure to detect this hepatitis and to stop the drug may result in cirrhosis.

The majority of drug hepatitis cases with symptoms present much like viral hepatitis, with nausea, vomiting, jaundice, and elevated liver enzymes. Symptoms usually appear within one to four weeks after the drug is started and disappear in about the same time when the drug is discontinued. Exceptions occur in drug allergy, which is mediated by the immune system. In these cases, symptoms begin immediately after exposure to the drug and are often accompanied by skin rash, usually due to inflammation of capillaries by an antigen-antibody reaction. Some drug reactions are predictably associated with liver tests that are characterized by damage to small bile ducts, poor bile drainage, and therefore elevated serum alkaline phosphatase levels with only minimal elevations of the level of serum enzymes; this is called cholestatic hepatitis and may take longer to disappear. Cholestatic reactions are characteristic of those associated with drugs prescribed for nausea but occur rarely.

If resolution does not occur within two to four weeks of stopping a suspect drug (with certain exceptions, such as some antiemetics and some drugs that are used in mental illness, it may take longer), there is considerable doubt that the drug is responsible for hepatitis. Death is a rare complication of these forms of drug hepatitis.

Idiosyncratic reactions tend to be severe, if discovery of the cause of the abnormal liver tests is delayed. Anticonvulsant drugs used in the treatment of epilepsy will occasionally cause this form of hepatitis, but, because this is well known, reactions are carefully watched for. On rare occasions such reactions occur only after several months of uncomplicated therapy.

Combinations of alcohol and acetaminophen markedly increase the toxicity of acetaminophen. Acetaminophen-induced hepatitis may occur with even normal doses, especially if taken daily. Serum ALT and AST levels characteristically begin to rise about forty-eight hours after ingestion. They may reach levels of 10,000 to 30,000 U/dL or higher but will fall within about seven days to near-normal levels if the dose was sublethal or treatment is prompt. Acute liver failure occurs with very large overdoses and with delayed treatment and may require liver transplantation for the patient's survival.

The major pathway by which drugs are detoxified in the liver is by glutathione, which liver cells normally contain in large amounts. If glutathione is depleted, as in alcoholism, prolonged fasting, or excess drug intake, metabolism of acetaminophen results in hepatotoxic compounds. Treatment consists of the removal of all acetaminophen remaining in the patient's gut by washing out the stomach with a tube passed through the nose. Absorption of any remaining drug can be inhibited by flushing charcoal through the tube. Additional cysteine that can be used to make new glutathione is supplied by putting a liquid compound called N-acetylcysteine (Mucomyst) through the tube into the gut. These treatment methods are highly effective if applied early.

Obviously, it is important for the physician to have a list of all drugs being taken by any patient with hepatitis. Prescription, over-the-counter (OTC) or nonprescription drugs, and herbal preparations should be included. Any drug started recently is especially suspect. The diagnosis of drug hepatitis is one of exclusion; that is, all known causes of viral or other forms of hepatitis are considered and ruled out through appropriate testing. Any newly started drug is immediately discontinued. Fortunately, drug hepatitis resolves in most cases when the offending agent is discontinued. Complete recovery means that the liver is normal in every way and no restrictions on other drugs are necessary.

Vitamin A

Vitamin A is hepatotoxic in large doses over long periods of time. It is present in OTC multivitamin preparations in concentrations as high as 25,000 IU. The recommended oral daily requirement is 5,000 IU, easily obtained in a normal diet. Retinol is vitamin A and is used in various skin diseases and to reduce wrinkles.

Vitamin A is stored in the liver in stellate cells that line the sinusoids (see chapter 1). Excessive amounts of this vitamin damage stellate cells, which are then transformed to cells that secrete fibrous tissue (see "cirrhosis" in chapter 2). Daily doses of greater than 10,000 IU may be hepatotoxic if taken over a long period of time. Liver injury has been described in those taking from 15,000 to 45,000 IU daily, and cirrhosis has been reported after intake of 25,000 every day for six years.

Herbs

The diversity of natural compounds is astounding. There are many weird and wonderful bioactive compounds that biochemists would never think of making. Unfortunately, the question of which ones are injurious and which ones are perhaps useful to humans requires careful study. Only a few of the ones that exist have been adequately evaluated.

It has only been within the past twenty-five years or so that we have learned enough about molecular configurations of disease-causing organisms, chemicals, and biological mechanisms to enable us to design unique drugs for the treatment of specific diseases. The progenitors of many of our present drugs were originally found in plants. The active ingredients were then purified, tested, and proven to be safe and effective. For example, the plant foxglove was a popular home remedy for "dropsy" (heart failure) in the eighteenth century. It was also known to be poisonous if given in large amounts. The active compound was subsequently named digitalis.

For centuries, bile harvested from bears was used as a home remedy for liver troubles in Asia. When studied, the active ingredient was identified as ursodeoxycholic acid, which is marketed today as Actigall or Ursodiol, a safe and effective treatment for certain kinds of chronic liver disease. Undoubtedly, some popular herbal remedies will prove to have useful ingredients, but many are already known to have dangerous properties as well. St. John's wort has recently been shown to interfere with metabolism of certain drugs used to prevent rejection in liver transplant patients, resulting in dangerously altered blood levels of those drugs. To date, careful scientific study has not been done on the vast majority of herbal remedies. Liver damage and hepatitis have been specifically noted in some, but the mechanism has not been clarified. One cannot assume that a remedy is innocuous just because it is a natural product, as opposed to being manufactured.

Milk thistle is probably the most widely used herbal preparation by patients with liver disease, including hepatitis C. It has been used in Asia for many decades and has been evaluated in clinical trials. The active ingredient is silymarin. This compound seems to be an antioxidant (like vitamin E) and may stabilize stellate cells. Administration of silymarin to patients with hepatitis C has resulted in some improvement in liver tests but has no effect on the virus of hepatitis C. No beneficial effects to long-term use have been demonstrated. No adverse reactions to the purified compound have been identified, but it damages cells in cell cultures.

Germander is used as a tea for weight loss and as a tonic. Several cases of severe hepatitis and fibrosis have been reported. Chaparral leaf, used as a general herbal remedy, causes a similar serious liver reaction. Oil of cloves is used for dental pain and is safe in small amounts used infrequently, but causes abnormal liver tests when taken chronically, as do mixed preparations containing mistletoe, skullcap, and valerian used as a laxative. A Chinese sedative and analgesic called Jin Bu Hunan anodyne tablets can cause severe hepatitis, fibrosis, and fatty liver. Because none of these has been systematically studied, the frequency of such adverse reactions is not known.

People generally are reluctant to confess to their physician that they are using herbal remedies. It is important for doctors to know that these preparations are being used when abnormal liver tests suggestive of hepatitis are found. Those who are on multiple prescriptions should not take herbal remedies simultaneously because of the possibility of converting safe drugs to unsafe ones.

Fatty Liver Hepatitis or Nonalcoholic Steatohepatitis (NASH Syndrome)

Accumulation of fat in the liver is the most common abnormality seen when a liver biopsy is examined microscopically and one of the most common causes of an enlarged liver. As a rule, fat is readily mobilized from the liver. It has traditionally been considered a completely benign abnormality, but in the past twenty years, an increasing number of cases have been found that have not been inconsequential.

We have been aware since antiquity that fat can engorge the liver. It is mentioned in several ancient manuscripts. With the development of the microscope and safe methods of biopsy, the histologic characteristics were further identified. Fatty liver is the earliest manifestation of heavy alcohol intake and disappears promptly if alcohol intake is stopped. It is commonly present in obese people, especially women, and in those with prolonged severe illness or protein malnutrition. Liver tests are normal in the majority of those with fatty liver.

Concern arose when it was found that infants and children in whom it was necessary to give all nutrition by vein and who developed a fatty liver regularly came to have cirrhosis. Adults treated in the same fashion often develop fatty liver but seldom cirrhosis. With refinements in methods of intravenous feeding, fatty liver now occurs infrequently. In the 1960s, when surgical operations were designed for the purpose of interfering with absorption of food as treatment for morbid obesity, many people undergoing those procedures developed fatty liver accompanied by hepatitis and the rapid onset of irreversible liver disease. However, when biopsies are performed on severely obese people before surgery, almost half are found to have a fatty liver, and, of these, at least mild-to-moderate fibrosis is present in about 70 percent, severe fibrosis in about 10 to 15 percent, and cirrhosis without any other known predisposing factor in 15 to 20 percent. Autopsy series show that cirrhosis is about six times more frequent in obese individuals than in those with normal amounts of body fat. The association between fatty liver and cirrhosis has only been recognized in the last twenty years.

By 1980, it was fully apparent that not all those with fatty liver have a benign course. It has long been recognized that diabetic patients commonly have fatty livers, with or without obesity, and that they have cirrhosis more frequently than nondiabetics, but obesity and cirrhosis were not previously known to be related. More aggressive investigations regarding obesity and diabetes, both separately and together, found that some had liver biopsies showing not only fat but also inflammation, or steatohepatitis ("steato-" is a Greek prefix referring to fat). Most of these biopsies came from individuals who had abnormal liver tests. Patients with fatty liver but no inflammation, or benign fatty liver, usually have normal liver tests. Under the microscope, steatohepatitis is indistinguishable from alcoholic hepatitis. Steatohepatitis is now called nonalcoholic steatohepatitis, or NASH syndrome. Biopsies over time show that those with NASH syndrome are at high risk for progression to cirrhosis.

It is difficult to estimate the prevalence of this syndrome, since liver biopsies are not routinely done on overweight or diabetic people. NASH syndrome probably accounts for many cases of cirrhosis without other known risk factors. Cirrhosis without any known cause is referred to as "cryptogenic." Suffice it to say that NASH syndrome is not uncommon.

The specific reasons for progression from fatty liver to hepatitis and thence to fibrosis and cirrhosis are unknown. While we can postulate many reasonable mechanisms, no single one explains all that we see. Our present knowledge thus suggests that a combination of many factors, including genetic ones, are involved; that is, the causes are probably multifactorial.

The typical patient with NASH syndrome is a middle-aged, obese female with type 2 diabetes (not requiring insulin) or with high levels of cholesterol (hypercholesterolemia) or of blood fats (hyperlipidemia). An enlarged liver is usually but not invariably present. Type 2 diabetes has developed in a few individuals after they have been found to have NASH syndrome. NASH syndrome has been present without any of these or other identifiable risk factors. It has been identified in children under the age of fifteen (as young as four), most of whom are obese and only a few of whom are diabetic. The condition has been associated with prolonged use of some drugs, such as cortisone compounds, heart medications (especially amiodarone), and lipid- and cholesterol-lowering drugs. It has been reported to occur more often in close relatives of patients with NASH syndrome than would be expected by chance alone, suggesting genetic involvement.

The majority with NASH syndrome have no symptoms, and the condition is discovered incidentally. A few will seek attention for vague intermittent pain over the liver or chronic fatigue. It can account for an enlarged liver of no known cause. It may also be responsible for mildly abnormal liver tests, with no other findings on physical examination. It should be suspected in all who have minor abnormalities in liver tests, especially in obese, diabetic females with an enlarged liver.

An enlarged liver may be the only abnormal finding on physical examination. The ALT and AST levels are mildly elevated in about 80 to 90 percent of patients. In contrast to the fatty liver of alcoholism, the serum ALT level is higher than the AST level. The alkaline phosphatase level is slightly to moderately elevated in about a third of patients. Total serum bilirubin and serum albumin levels are normal until cirrhosis is present. A sonogram or CT scan may suggest a fatty liver, whereas the more expensive magnetic resonance image (MRI) shows a characteristic "bright" liver if fat is present. An elevated blood sugar, cholesterol, or blood fat (lipids/triglycerides) level may be present and identifies the risk factors.

Diagnosis of NASH syndrome is accomplished through ruling out all other forms of hepatitis by the taking of a careful history and the performing of laboratory studies. A liver biopsy is usually diagnostic and advisable in most suspected cases, but is not recommended for those with a fatty liver and persistently normal liver tests. Biopsy shows not only fat and inflammatory cells but evidence of cell death and fibrosis. Alcoholic hyaline, or Mallory bodies, may be present, and so may fully developed and previously unsuspected cirrhosis.

Treatment of NASH involves treatment or control of any identified associated disease. Low-fat diets, weight loss, control of diabetes, and treatment of high blood cholesterol or high blood fat levels are fundamental. It is not yet clear that such efforts are efficacious in reversing the changes in the liver. Drugs, including those purchased over the counter, as well as herbal remedies, should be discontinued if possible. Many of these recommendations are difficult to carry out over a lifetime.

The use of the synthetic bile acid called ursodeoxycholic acid (Actigall or Ursodiol), is associated with mobilization of liver fat. Initial therapeutic trials have given encouraging results but no proof that it prevents progression to cirrhosis. This synthetic bile is largely without side effects, although a few people will have mild diarrhea, and its use has become common. Liver transplantation may be required for advanced NASH syndrome with cirrhosis.

Immune Hepatitis

An autoimmune disease is one that results from the development of antibodies that are directed against one's own body tissues. Such diseases occur usually without known provocation, are persistent (that is, chronic), and are characterized by marked inflammatory reactions in and destruction of the effected tissue. Rheumatoid arthritis and lupus are perhaps the best known of these diseases.

There are several autoimmune diseases of the liver, but only one is commonly referred to as autoimmune hepatitis. Brief discussions of two additional ones, primary biliary cirrhosis (PBC) and primary sclerosing cholangitis (PSC), are worth including here because both are fairly common and are autoimmune diseases, and because chronic hepatitis that progresses to cirrhosis is present in both. These three diseases involve (1) hepatic cells, (2) smallest bile ducts, and (3) larger bile ducts, respectively.

In autoimmune diseases, including those of the liver, multiple antibodies are often present in serum that do not seem to be in any way related to the primary problem, such as antithyroid antibodies and antibodies against acid-secreting cells of the stomach. Others are so consistently present that they are used as markers of the disease (but are not the cause of it). For example, antinuclear antibodies, directed against proteins found in all cell nuclei, are useful markers of a number of autoimmune diseases, including autoimmune hepatitis. All other forms of hepatitis must be ruled out in suspected cases.

The prevalence of immune hepatitis is unknown because it is so commonly without symptoms and is found only incidentally in routine examinations for unrelated reasons. Therefore, we do not know how many people have it. Suffice it to say that it is not uncommon.

Autoimmune hepatitis (AIH) has been classified into three types. By far the most common in this country is type I, often referred to as "classic" AIH. About 80 percent of cases occur in young women with a mean age of forty (+ fifteen) years, but it may be seen in older women. Why a smaller proportion of males have the disease is unknown but is in keeping with the pattern in many other, nonhepatic, autoimmune diseases. Even in asymptomatic and apparently healthy people with AIH, ALT and AST levels are markedly elevated, commonly in the range of 500 to 1,000 U/dL (normal being less than

45 or 70, depending upon the laboratory instrument used).
Serum gammaglobulin levels are typically elevated. Serum
antinuclear antibodies (ANA) are present in about 90 percent
and anti—smooth muscle antibodies in about 60 percent.
Liver biopsy shows inflammatory cells with a single, well-
formed nucleus in the area where the smallest branches of the
portal vein and hepatic artery enter the liver lobule and small
bile ducts leave (the portal area) (see fig. 1.3). In the more
severe cases, inflammatory cells extend into the liver lobule.
Some degree of fibrosis is always present, and many patients
have fully developed cirrhosis at the time of discovery.

About 40 percent of patients with type 1 AIH have other
autoimmune diseases concurrently, such as autoimmune thyroiditis, chronic ulcerative colitis, rheumatoid arthritis, various forms of autoimmune anemia, inflammation of small
blood vessels in the skin (vasculitis), nephritis, and fibrosis
in the lung.

A genetic component is involved in autoimmune liver
disease. It frequently occurs in first-degree relatives of patients, such as mother-daughter or sister-sister tandem, and
antibodies seen in this disease may also be found in first-
degree relatives without this or other disease. Moreover, it
has a higher incidence in identical than in fraternal twins. It
is not inherited in the usual sense; that is, it is not predictable
and does not follow recognized rules of inheritance.

Because there is often considerable overlapping of signs,
symptoms, and laboratory tests in the several forms of immune hepatitis, it is sometimes difficult to definitively assign
a specific disease entity to an individual. This is often the
case in patients who have features of both AIH and PBC, a
situation that is referred to as "overlap" syndrome.

Type 2 AIH is uncommon in this country. It occurs in
adults and in children aged two to fifteen years, but the latter
make up only about 4 percent of cases of type 2 AIH in
the United States (compared to over 25 percent of those in
Europe). Clinically, it is similar to "classical" type 1 but has

antibodies that cross-react with liver, kidney, and microsomal proteins (anti-LKM). It has the same natural history as type I and responds to treatment similarly.

Type 3 AIH is rare. It is marked by antibodies that are specifically directed against liver-membrane antigen (SLA). SLA is not available in hospital laboratories.

The natural history of untreated AIH is one of slow progression to cirrhosis over a period of ten to twenty years or longer. It should be noted here that since this disease is most often seen in young women of childbearing age, pregnancy is safe and not contraindicated. Some patients never reach the stage of cirrhosis, although the number is probably small. Without treatment, liver tests are persistently abnormal as described above. For those in whom the diagnosis is made late in the course and irreversible cirrhosis has developed or treatment fails, liver transplantation is commonly required. Unfortunately, the disease sometimes recurs in the transplanted liver.

On rare occasions, AIH may appear rather suddenly and progress rapidly. These forms are difficult to differentiate from other forms of acute hepatitis and may rapidly progress to cirrhosis. Response to treatment in such patients is more often unsatisfactory.

Remission of the disease and prevention of cirrhosis is attained in about 85 percent of patients through use of corticosteroids (prednisone). Remission can be maintained by the immunosuppressant drug azathioprine (Imuran) or by often remarkably small doses of prednisone. Relapse occurs within six months in more than half of patients if treatment is stopped. Because prolonged use of corticosteroids causes osteoporosis, cataracts, and occasionally a fatty liver, azathioprine is preferable in maintaining remission. The initial concern that azathioprine might be associated with development of malignancies appears unfounded.

Primary biliary cirrhosis (PBC) is a form of autoimmune hepatitis in which the target of the attack is not hepatic cells but the smallest bile ducts. Destruction of these small ducts causes interference with secretion and drainage of bile, followed by hepatitis, leading eventually to cirrhosis. PBC is a misnomer when applied to the early stage of the disease because in most cases the diagnosis is made well before cirrhosis appears. Although we continue to refer to "PBC," the more appropriate term for the precirrhotic stage is chronic nonsuppurative cholangitis.

As in other autoimmune diseases of the liver, PBC progresses slowly over a period of years. It tends to develop in stepwise fashion, remaining stable for long but variable periods (at least months and often years) only to become worse over a relatively short period and then become stable again. The disease is asymptomatic early in its course. The most common first symptom is generalized itching; it is due to retention of bile in the skin and can be intense. It is usually accompanied by elevated levels of serum bile acids that cannot be secreted through the damaged bile ducts. Because cholesterol also cannot be excreted normally, it tends to accumulate and form deposits in the skin, especially around the eyes and elbows. These are known as xanthalasma. A common accompanying symptom is dryness of the mouth and eyes, caused by immunological damage to salivary and tear glands. This is the sicca or Sjögren's syndrome. Pain may result from microfractures of bone due to a secondary defect in vitamin D metabolism, causing abnormal utilization of calcium. As in type i AIH, there may be thyroiditis or other immune-associated diseases. Cirrhosis develops after fifteen to thirty years and often requires liver transplantation. Recurrence of PBC in the transplanted liver has been seen.

The diagnosis of PBC is made by finding the characteristic antibodies in the serum and examining liver tissue obtained by biopsy. The antibody that characterizes PBC is directed toward the inner membrane of mitochondria of the hepatic cell and is called the antimitochondrial antibody. (Mitochondria are round structures in the cytoplasm of every cell that produce energy for the cell from carbohydrates, fats, and proteins.) It is present in approximately 90 percent of cases of PBC but may be seen in other diseases as well; that is, it is not specific for PBC. Abnormal liver tests consist of mild-to-moderate elevations of ALT and AST but marked elevation of serum alkaline phosphatase levels, reflecting interference with bile drainage. This pattern is also seen in other forms of obstruction to bile flow, and these must be ruled out when PBC is considered. Cholesterol and lipids cannot be secreted normally for the same reason and accumulate in the blood. Serum gammaglobulin levels are variably elevated. In PBC, it is the IgM type that are characteristically (but not invariably) increased. In this disease, the IgM globulins never become IgG type, as is true in infectious diseases. Serum bilirubin is not elevated until late in the disease.

Liver biopsy is often necessary to differentiate this disease from several others that can be accompanied by similar liver test abnormalities. The destruction of small bile ducts can be recognized under the microscope, as can other findings associated with this disease. Fibrosis is present in variable amounts. Cirrhosis may be present when PBC is first discovered.

Unfortunately, treatment of PBC is not satisfactory. Corticosteroids and azathioprine have been prospectively evaluated and found to have little effect. The former worsens the bone disease known to be present and thus is not used. Another drug that suppresses the immune system, methotrexate, has been used in an experimental setting with only moderate and largely unsatisfactory effectiveness. At the present time, it appears that only the synthetic bile acid ursodeoxycholic acid (Actigall or Ursodiol) delays progression of this disease. It is given as tablets in divided doses for a total dose of 900 to 1000 mg. per day. Vitamin D and calcium supplements are advisable, because, in this disease and for unclear reasons, the metabolism of ingested vitamin D by the diseased liver is deficient. It has been observed that the resulting bone disease seen in PBC can be prevented by ingestion of this vitamin.

Prognosis of PBC varies. Some patients never develop cirrhosis, while in others it progresses relatively rapidly. Liver tests are closely monitored. When the serum bilirubin becomes elevated and is consistently above a level of 3 mg/dL, evaluation for liver transplantation is recommended.

Primary sclerosing cholangitis (PSC) is considered to be another form of autoimmune hepatitis of the liver, although the underlying mechanism has not been definitively identified. It is characterized by inflammation in multiple scattered areas of larger bile ducts, in contrast to PBC, in which the smallest ducts are attacked. The ducts are those large enough to be seen with the unaided eye. This process causes fibrosis of the ducts, resulting in narrowed areas (strictures) through which bile cannot pass. Inflammation of the liver is secondary to obstruction of bile flow. Cirrhosis develops slowly over a period of years.

There are several other forms of sclerosing cholangitis, which therefore represents a spectrum of diseases. Discussion of these other forms, usually a feature of recognized systemic disease, is beyond the scope of this book, but the most common association is with another autoimmune disease, chronic ulcerative colitis. About 60 to 80 percent of those with PSC have this disease, usually for several years before the appearance of PSC. On the other hand, ulcerative colitis may be found only after PSC is discovered. Approximately 2 to 5 percent of those with ulcerative colitis develop PSC.

Primary carcinoma of the bile ducts (cholangiocarcinoma) looks a great deal like PSC and is therefore difficult to differentiate from it, even in the most experienced hands. This form of malignancy can develop in patients who have had PSC for several years, further confounding the diagnosis.

In contrast in AIH and PBC, no recognized antibodies are present in PSC. Antinuclear, antimitochondrial and anti— smooth muscle antibodies are absent. Although the diagnosis may be suggested by liver biopsy, it is usually not diagnostic. Studies that visualize the bile ducts are necessary and usually definitive. The procedure most often used is endoscopic retrograde cholangiopancreatography, or ERCP. In this procedure, the patient is put under sedation and a flexible instrument is introduced through the mouth and stomach into the upper small intestine to allow visualization of the opening of the common bile duct into the gut. A small plastic tube is passed through a channel in the instrument and inserted into the duct. A liquid contrast material is injected to fill the ducts. This material can be seen under the fluoroscope, and strictures or irregularities can be identified. Characteristic strictures in multiple areas of the ducts confirm the diagnosis. Magnetic resonance cholangiopancreatography, or MRCP, a special form of magnetic resonance imaging (MRI), is a rapidly developing technique that also allows visualization of the large ducts without the need for introduction of a tube. It is not yet widely available.

There is no satisfactory treatment of PSC at present. If a single stricture is dominant, it can be dilated by the placing and inflation of a collapsed balloon within the stricture. Unfortunately, such an isolated stricture is not common. Ursodeoxycholic acid, discussed above under treatment of PBC, may be helpful but does not change the slowly progressive nature of the disease. PSC is a common reason for liver transplantation.

Bacterial Hepatitis

Small numbers of bacteria normally gain access to the bloodstream during such mundane daily activities as brushing one's teeth. Bacteria in the blood without disease is called bacteremia. An important normal function of the liver is to help remove these bacteria. In the event of serious infections anywhere in the body, the number of bacteria that enter the circulation may be very large and may overwhelm many defensive mechanisms. Such an event is extremely serious and is referred to as sepsis. Sepsis commonly causes abnormal liver tests through products of inflammation without actual infection in the liver itself. In other words, the liver is participating in the generalized reaction induced by sepsis. Occasionally, however, bacteria may actually infect the liver, causing hepatitis or even abscess formation.

A good example of bacterial hepatitis is that which occurs relatively frequently in severe pneumonia. Liver biopsy reveals bacteria and inflammatory cells within the liver tissue. When the source of the bacteria is the colon, abscesses within the liver may occur. Now that we have much more effective antibiotics, such occurrences are relatively uncommon.

Bacteria produce toxins as by-products of their metabolism. In addition, destruction of bacteria result in degradation of bacterial cell walls which may themselves be toxins. Bacterial toxins stimulate the release of cytokines and directly inhibit normal hepatic function. One of the most common manifestations of sepsis is low serum albumin levels. This occurs because the messenger RNA in the liver that directs albumin synthesis is strongly inhibited by bacterial toxins. Albumin production virtually stops. Probably the second most common effect of toxins is interference with the metabolism and secretion of bile into bile ducts, mimicking mechanical obstruction, which must be ruled out. Serum alkaline phosphatase (see chapter I) levels become elevated, and serum bilirubin levels rise above normal levels. Mild jaundice is common.

Bacterial hepatitis is treated by antibiotics directed at the primary source of infection. It usually resolves promptly but reflects bacterial infection somewhere in the body that may result in death. Liver abscesses usually require drainage by needle puncture in addition to antibiotics.

Other infectious organisms may directly involve the liver just as they do any other portion of the body. These include the spirochete that causes syphilis, some fungi, and several kinds of parasites. Amoebic dysentery, now seen infrequently in the United States but still common in Mexico, South America, and other countries, is commonly accompanied by abscesses of the liver. Amoebic abscess responds rapidly to needle drainage and to an antibiotic called metronidazole (Flagyl).

7. Current Research

Genetic Engineering

Efforts to manipulate the genetic structure of the hepatitis viruses with the goal of preventing their reproduction have met with limited but encouraging success. One type of investigation binds complementary ("antisense") nucleotides to portions of the viral genes. Antisense nucleotides are those that bind to a target gene and prevent a function because it cannot be interpreted by the metabolic processes of the virus, which cannot then reproduce. Such disabled viruses might be useful in inducing neutralizing (protective) antibodies. If we can discover a way to bind such antisense segments to the genes of virus infecting an individual, the disease can be cured. Much more of this research must be done before it can be applied to humans.

One of the essential steps in infection of cells by any virus is attachment to specific receptors on the liver cell surface followed by entry into the cell (see chapter 1). If these receptors can be thoroughly characterized, it is possible that innocuous compounds can be formulated which occupy them, therefore making them unavailable to the virus. Research in this area continues but is not close to being available for human application.

Prevention

Few research efforts are being made to develop additional vaccines against hepatitis A and B, because those we have are so effective. Presently available vaccines against HAV are 98 to 100 percent effective in inducing protective antibodies against the disease. While it is possible to virtually eliminate this disease, current vaccines are too expensive for widespread use in those countries that are reservoirs for this disease.

The vaccines presently in use to prevent HBV are safe and effective in 90 to 95 percent of those who receive the recommended doses. This vaccine is presently produced by recombinant technology, as described in chapter 4.

Efforts to develop a vaccine against HCV have been disappointing. No vaccine is currently available. The difficulty arises from the rapid mutation of the virus in portions of its structure that would normally serve as the focus of vaccine development. In addition, there is no widely available tissue culture system satisfactory for study of those elements necessary for the development of an effective vaccine. Early vaccines tested in chimpanzees provided only partial and short-lived protection. Since present tests for antibodies in hepatitis C identify only the nonneutralizing (that is, nonprotective) antibodies, efforts continue to identify antibodies that reflect immunity. It is known that about 15 to 25 percent of people infected with HCV obliterate the virus, apparently doing so through complex interaction of several arms of the immune system, including protective neutralizing antibodies and sensitized T cells. Further study of the immune mechanisms of those few who spontaneously eliminate the virus may allow the development of an effective vaccine.

A promising approach to HCV vaccine development has involved investigations into a DNA-based vaccine by means of one of several methods. It is possible to extract from the HCV gene small segments of its RNA that are essential to its survival. These segments can be combined with DNA made in the laboratory and directly injected intramuscularly into mice, which develop antibodies against the RNA; presumably, these antibodies would be effective against the virus in humans. Studies in nonhuman primates have not yet been reported. A second "DNA vaccine" is being studied in which similar vital segments of HCV RNA are inserted into the genes of benign viruses and injected into animals. Antibodies develop against HCV; further, T lymphocytes that appear to be cytotoxic develop in this preparation. Other approaches, including the injection of short segments of the HCV gene isolated from essential RNA segments (making it noninfectious), are also being attempted. It is to be emphasized that none of these vaccines has been shown to neutralize the naturally occurring virus, but the experiments offer hope for a safe and effective vaccine against hepatitis C in the future.

New Drug Treatments

Treatment of acute infection with any virus is hampered by the resistance of viruses to most known drugs that are not prohibitively injurious to the patient. Research efforts to find such drugs have had limited success. Since most of the hepatitis viruses reproduce and are transmitted to others before disease is recognized, and since the disease is usually self-limited, such drugs would have little usefulness in acute cases. They would, however, be useful in preventing persistent infection that leads to chronic disease.

Given the situation in treatment of HIV, the AIDS virus, it is generally agreed among investigators that three or more simultaneously used drugs would probably be required in order to eliminate HCV at a reasonable rate. Such combinations of drugs have resulted in a significant increase in response rates in HIV disease.

Blood levels of interferon α become lower than detectable eight to twelve hours after each injection. The number of HCV viral RNA particles in serum falls precipitously when interferon α levels are high but rapidly rises as interferon α levels fall. When interferon α is again injected forty-eight hours after the first dose, the number of viral particles has again attained its original level. Persistent suppression of viral reproduction is achieved by sustained levels of interferon α, but the necessity of several injections each day to attain these levels of drug is impractical. A new form of interferon called "pegylated interferon" will soon be on the market, the chief advantage of which is that it requires one injection per week. This drug is interferon α in which a molecule of polyethylene glycol has been inserted. The drug is slowly absorbed, sustaining a consistently high blood level of interferon α over time. With this form of interferon α, serum viral levels are persistently suppressed. The use of pegylated interferon as monotherapy for forty-eight weeks results in sustained elimination of the HCV virus at nearly the same rate as the combination of interferon α given three times a week plus ribavirin tablets taken daily for forty-eight weeks. The side effects of interferon α and of its pegylated form are essentially identical. In several large trials currently under way, dual therapy with pegylated interferon plus ribavirin is being tested. At least theoretically, this form of therapy should be superior to the non—pegylated interferon plus ribavirin therapy currently in use.

Additional trials of interferon treatment include induction therapy, in which large doses are given on a daily basis followed by smaller doses three times a week for forty-eight weeks, continuous daily doses, larger doses, or intravenous infusions. These efforts are experimental and not customarily used outside of research protocols. At this point it is not clear that any of these methods is significantly more effective than those that are recommended and commonly used.

Ongoing trials involve testing the feasibility of giving interferon α three times every week over a period of years to those who have failed to eliminate the virus after conventional periods. Preliminary data suggest that it is possible to continuously suppress the virus and avoid ongoing liver damage. The major disadvantage, of course, is the necessity for regular injections over years and the persistent side effects of this drug.

Readers interested in entering clinical trials should call their nearest medical school or contact the National Institutes of Health, which maintains a list of such protocals (see appendix).

The FDA-approved drugs amantadine and rimantadine, useful in influenza A and some other viral diseases, have been tried as single agents in HCV protocols and found to be ineffective. Initial studies indicate that, when these drugs are used in combination with interferon and ribavirin (triple drug therapy), there is a higher response rate as measured by improvement in liver tests and in suppression of the virus than when interferon and ribavirin are used as double drug therapy. More studies will be required to clearly indicate if we should routinely use either of these drugs in a triple therapy strategy.

Glycyrrhizin, like milk thistle (silymarin) a popular treatment of chronic liver disease in Japan for decades, has been tested and found to have no effect on the HCV virus but does tend to cause lowering of the serum ALT. A trial using glycyrrhizin in combination with ursodeoxycholic acid found effects similar to those when each was used alone; i.e., there was no effect on the virus but there was a significant lowering of ALT levels that did not persist after the drugs were discontinued.

Trials in which injections of the cytokines interleukin-6, interleukin-10, and interleukin-12 are used have tended to be associated with diminution in serum ALT levels but with little or no effect on the virus levels. These results are reminiscent of the effect of ribavirin when used as monotherapy. No trial of interleukin therapy in combination with interferon or other drugs has been published, but this remains an attractive possible approach.

We do not yet have a satisfactory treatment of primary biliary cirrhosis, which remains one of the frequent causes of liver transplant. Methotrexate, also used in other autoimmune diseases, continues to be the object of clinical trials either as a single drug or in combination with others. Results have been encouraging but not definitive, and methotrexate is still considered an experimental treatment of primary biliary cirrhosis.

Artificial Liver Support Systems

Some exciting work is being done that makes hepatic cells available to the acutely failing liver or involves replacing destroyed cells without transplanting a whole organ. While many of these investigations are several years away from application, a few may be useful within the next five years.

In desperate attempts to save the lives of people who were dying of acute liver failure, cross perfusion of blood between patients and animals or other humans were performed on several occasions in the past. The animals were pigs or chimpanzees. Patient improvement was definite and transient, but these efforts did demonstrate that perfusion of blood through a healthy liver, even across species, worked temporarily, and encouraged continued efforts. In addition to obvious ethical concerns, there were many technical problems, such as clotting of blood in the connecting tubes, destruction of platelets, causing bleeding, and allergic reactions to the donor liver (hyperacute rejection). Cross perfusion has not been done since the late 1950s.

Whole livers from pigs, chimpanzees, and humans recently deceased have also been attached to blood vessels outside of patients in extracorporeal experiments, attempts to substitute for the sick liver. In these efforts, the time of perfusion is limited to two to six hours before the donor liver begins to deteriorate and fails to function. This failure is probably the result of a lack of arterial blood flow. During the brief time of perfusion, some improvement in patients has been seen in brain function and lowering of the serum bilirubin levels, but there is no lasting benefit. The current success with human-to-human liver transplantation raises the cogent argument that any available liver should be transplanted rather than used for only a few hours. Whole organ perfusion has also been abandoned.

Stimulated by the partial success of whole organ perfusion, efforts are under way to incorporate living hepatic cells into various devices, or "artificial livers," with encouraging results in the several cases in which they have been used. At least four companies are actively pursuing development of an artificial liver. Only recently has any such device been subjected to rigorous clinical trials. Both human and pig liver cells have been used. The pig is a favorite choice for use either in these efforts or in those using whole organs that have been genetically altered so that they will be more compatible with human tissue (see below). The size of the pig liver is similar to that of humans, and its harvested cells withstand the rigors of isolation and tissue culture better than those of other animals. In these devices, tiny porous tubes or special membranes separate the liver cells from blood or plasma pumped over them, yet allow exchange of proteins and other vital materials synthesized by the cells. At the moment, the most successful arrangement has been one in which pig liver cells are cultured and grow in the tubes or on membranes before use, allowing a large increase in the number of functioning cells. Since pig cells produce pig protein, antibodies are formed in the patient and can damage pig cells used in subsequent perfusion treatments. These devices can operate effectively for several hours and be replaced by newly produced ones. Theoretically, it would be best to mimic an intact liver by continuous perfusion of blood or plasma. However, preliminary studies suggest that discontinuous use, such as eight to twelve hours per day, accomplishes almost as much as attempts to perfuse continuously and at substantially less effort and expense.

These "artificial livers" hold considerable promise. They have been classified as drugs by the FDA because the pig cells could release unknown substances into the blood. As drugs, they must pass a number of tests, going through ran-

domized, controlled trials before they can be widely used.
There is, for example, concern that animal viruses contained
in the cells may gain access to humans and even be transmitted to others with potentially disastrous results. In trials to
date, no such transmission has been recognized.

Treatment of acute liver failure with the use of artificial
kidney machines has been tried but provides no benefit.
The artificial kidney is highly effective in substituting for the
kidneys, but cannot substitute for multiple vital functions of
the liver.

Liver and Liver Cell Transplantation

Long-term survival rates after liver transplantation have
continued to improve. The overall five-year survival rate is
now around 85 to 90 percent. In a number of cases, not
only the liver but also the pancreas or kidneys have been
simultaneously transplanted. Livers transplanted into patients
who have chronic hepatitis B or C acquire the disease in all
cases. Drugs which would occupy the receptor proteins on
liver cells and thus prevent such infection, as discussed above,
would be an attractive strategy if such drugs can be found
and shown to be safe. Efforts to ameliorate posttransplant
infection with prophylactic lamivudine (hepatitis B) or inter-
feron/ribavirin (hepatitis C) continue with moderate success.
As a rule the disease is suppressed by antirejection drugs, and
overt clinical disease is delayed for some years.

Efforts to transplant only portions of liver from living
donors or from one cadaver liver into more than one recipient
(split-liver transplantation) have been variably successful.
When used in patients with acute hepatitis, successful transplants function until the injured liver recovers, at which point
the grafted liver becomes atrophic and antirejection medica-
tion can be discontinued. This technique addresses in part the
problem of a shortage of livers suitable for transplantation,

and the results to date suggest that it will be used more often in the future. The surgical technique is demanding. The liver has a complex vascular structure. Dividing it during an operation requires special skills so that vessels in the remaining liver will not be injured and to insure that the donor has sufficient liver for survival. While the risk to the living donor is appreciable, the mortality rate of the operation is less than 3 percent.

In experimental animals, liver cell transplantation has shown promising results. In this procedure, liver cells from donor animals are harvested and injected into the portal vein of the recipient. They lodge in the liver, where they grow and function normally. In a recent experiment, liver cells from mice were harvested, processed, and deep-frozen. After several days, the cells were thawed and tested for viability. Cell survival has varied from 10 to 80 percent in different preparations. More important, with proper handling these cells retain their ability to regenerate. In one report, an injection of hepatic cells equivalent to 0.1 percent of the mass of the animal's liver not only survived but regenerated a liver mass equivalent to about 30 percent of the original mass. That is enough liver mass to insure survival of the individual when it is combined with the original liver. If this procedure can be reproduced in human subjects, it holds a great deal of promise. In acute fulminant hepatitis with liver failure, the life of the patient will be prolonged, giving time for the sick liver to regenerate. The procedure has the potential for taking the place of whole organ transplants at a much lower cost. For those with chronic liver disease who are not candidates for whole organ transplants, it could be life saving.

Current research in manipulating stem cells to grow new livers holds tremendous potential for replacement of diseased livers. It is likely that stem cells, especially if they can be isolated from the individuals into whom they will be inserted, will be the best source for hepatic cell transplantation as described in the previous chapter. Certainly, it will be many years before this technique will be available for common use.

Pigs that are given human genes for production of human protein are a potential source of livers that are largely indistinguishable from those of humans. Once engineered, these pigs can be bred or cloned to produce a large supply of organs of several kinds. Sufficient investigation of the tolerance of another species for such genetically engineered organs has not yet been done. If a large number of such animals become available and the livers from them are as well tolerated as projected, the present shortage of livers for transplantation would be solved. A concern yet to be adequately resolved is the possibility that animal viruses not now transmissible to humans will be implanted along with the organs and that these viruses may prove to cause disease and could even be passed to other individuals. We have used processed pig heart valves for several years with no evidence of disease to date, but this does not obviate the concern. It has recently been reported that analysis of the genetic structure of humans and animals alike indicates that fragments resembling those of viruses are already present in both.

While there are ethical objections to this procedure by animal activists, I can't believe that children and adults will be allowed to die in order to preserve the lives of pigs. It remains to be proven, however, that such manipulation of animal genes will, in fact, produce livers immunologically and physiologically indistinguishable from those of humans.

In summary, we can say that cases of hepatitis caused by viruses and those resulting from ingestion of toxic substances are still common throughout the world, and that they are serious and sometimes have life-threatening consequences, but that acute cases are not usually fatal. Some, especially hepatitis C, are dangerous either because, once they are acquired, we have difficulty getting rid of them, or because we don't recognize the problem until irreversible damage has occurred. The disease may therefore be chronic and cause persistent inflammation, with cirrhosis developing as an end result. The majority of hepatitis cases caused by viruses are preventable. We have highly effective vaccines against two of the three most common types caused by viruses (hepatitis A and B) and reason to hope that at some point there will be one against the third (hepatitis C). As sanitation improves around the world, the prevalence of cases with viral causes will diminish, but we must continue to be cautious with new drugs for treatment of other diseases to prevent (or at least recognize early) liver disease secondary to them. Our treatments of both acute and chronic hepatitis leave much to be desired, but current research promises better results in the future. As our ability to manipulate the genetic structure of all organisms advances, we will develop new treatments and, along the way, will have to answer serious ethical questions, but we have reason to be optimistic. According to a well-established axiom, knowledge brings power over our afflictions, and, equally important, gives us some peace of mind. It is as true with hepatitis as with any other disease.

Appendix

Further Reading

Di Bisceglie, Adrian M., M.D., and Bruce R. Bacon, M.D. "The Unmet Challenges of Hepatitis C." *Scientific American* (October 1999): 81–85.

Organizations

The American Liver Foundation
1425 Pompton Ave.
Cedar Grove, NJ 07009–1000
800–223-0179
(See Online Services below.)

Hepatitis Foundation International
30 Sunrise Terrace
Cedar Grove, NJ 07009–1423
800–891-0707

NDDIC
2 Information Way
Bethesda, MD 20892–3570
301–654-3810

Online Services

National Institutes of Health (patient information)
www.nlm.nih.gov/medlineplus

American Liver Foundation (patient information materials)
www.liverfoundation.org
800–223-0179

Hepatitis B Foundation (patient information on all aspects of hepatitis B)
www.hepb.org

Hepatitis Foundation International (multilingual; hepatitis A—E)
www.hepfi.org

Centers for Disease Control and Prevention
www.cdc.gov/hepatitis

See also:
www.HepWeb
www.HepNet

Assistance Programs

The following programs help uninsured or underinsured patients obtain financial coverage for medications used in the treatment of hepatitis C. Interested persons will need to provide their doctor's name and address and their diagnosis and prescription. Those who have insurance will be asked for their policy number as well as their insurance company's address and phone number.

Schering-Plough Corp. (makers of Intron A(R) alpha-interferon and Rebetron(R) combination of interferon and ribavirin). *Commitment to Care.* 800–521-7157.

Roche Laboratories (makers of Roferon(R) interferon-2a). *HepLine.* 800–443-6676.

Amgen (makers of consensus interferon). *Safety Net.* 888–508-8088.

Glossary

Albumin A necessary protein in the body; produced only by the liver. Albumin is a carrier protein that transports small compounds throughout the body. It adds to the osmotic pressure in blood, which maintains water in the circulation.

ALT (alanine transaminase) An enzyme produced by hepatic cells. Normally, some leaks into serum; when the cell membrane is injured, a great deal more crosses into serum. ALT is often measured to determine whether hepatic cells are injured.

Anemia A state of having too little hemoglobin in the blood.

Anorexia Loss of appetite.

Antibody A form of immune globulin produced by specialized B cells after stimulation by an antigen. Each acts specifically against the antigen in an immune response.

Antiemetic A drug that combats nausea and vomiting.

Antigen A protein or carbohydrate substance (such as a toxin or enzyme) capable of stimulating an immune response (see antibody). A protein that is not recognized as a part of the body (not "self") acts as an antigen.

Ascites Fluid in the cavity of the abdomen. It is common in advanced liver disease and occurs in other diseases as well.

AST (aspartate transaminase) An enzyme made in the liver and in many other organs.

Asterixis The inability to maintain a sustained muscle contraction. For instance, a "flap" of the hand at the wrist occurs when a patient tries to keep the hand extended. Asterixis is a sign of impending liver coma.

Asymptomatic Without symptoms.

Atrophy Shrinkage with loss of function.

Autoantibodies Antibodies that have been formed against body tissues. The immune system no longer recognizes these tissues as part of "self" and reacts to them as foreign.

Bacteremia Bacteria in the blood. Usually transient, this is a common condition in healthy people.

Bilirubin A yellow pigment metabolized by the liver that is the normal end product of hemoglobin breakdown. When it accumulates in tissues, as in liver disease, it is recognized as jaundice.

Biopsy The removal and examination of tissue from the living body.

Caput medusae A tangle of enlarged veins around the umbilicus. These veins are connected to the portal system as the residua of the vein connecting the fetus to the placenta. The condition reflects portal hypertension.

Carcinoma Malignancy (cancer) of epithelial cells that can originate in many tissue types.

Catalyze To cause a reaction to occur more rapidly.

Cholangitis Inflammation of bile ducts.

Cirrhosis An advanced stage of scarring (fibrosis) of the liver.

Coagulate To clot or congeal.

Collagen A type of fibrous protein that is present in all tissue; the major protein of scar tissue.

CT (computed tomography) The technique of taking multiple x rays through a specific area and reconstructing a radiographic picture with a computer. The result is a cross section x-ray picture of the area.

Cytokines Messenger proteins of the immune system that signal cells to react in a way that is specific to the target cell. Cytokines are released as a part of the inflammatory process and may either cause additional inflammation or inhibit it.

Cytopathic Causing damage to or destruction of cells.

Dehydration A deficiency of water.

Diaphragm Two large flat and domed muscles, right and left, that separate the chest cavities from the abdominal cavity. When they contract, they flatten and make for a larger chest cavity, drawing air into the lungs and pushing down on the liver.

dL (deciliter) In the metric system, one-tenth of a liter; a hundred milliliters. **Edema** Excessive water in tissue.

Emesis The act of vomiting.

Encephalopathy Dysfunction of the brain caused by metabolic or structural disturbances. The condition is characterized by confusion, disorientation, and, when severe, coma.

Endemic Prevalent in or characteristic of a population or region.

Endoscope A long flexible instrument with either optical fibers or light-sensitive computer chips that transmit a picture to a TV monitor, thus allowing visualization of internal organs.

Fibrosis Scar tissue (see collagen).

Gluconeogenesis Generation of glucose by the liver from proteins and non-glucose carbohydrates.

Glucose The most elementary form of sugar. Carbohydrates must be in the form of glucose or closely related sugars in order to move across most cell membranes and into the cell.

Glycogen A complex of multiple molecules of glucose. This form can be stored and later reduced to glucose for use by cells.

Gynecomastia Abnormal enlargement of the breasts; usually applied to males.

Hemoglobin The protein in red blood cells that carries oxygen. When red blood cells are senescent or destroyed by disease, bilirubin is formed.

Hemorrhage Bleeding.

Hepatic Pertaining to the liver.

Hepatic artery Along with the portal vein, one of the two blood suppliers to the liver; provides highly oxygenated blood to hepatic cells.

Hepatitis Inflammation of the liver.

Hepatomegaly Enlargement of the liver.

Hepatotoxic Toxic or poisonous to the liver; related to or causing injury to the liver.

Hepatotrophic Growing and reproducing primarily in the liver.

Histology The study of cells as they appear under the microscope; tissue structure or organization.

HIV Human immunovirus, the cause of AIDS. It selectively destroys T cells and thus severely inhibits the immune system.

Homeostasis A stable state of equilibrium among the elements of a system.

Hyperlipemia Abnormally high levels of fat (lipid) in the blood; same as hyperlipidemia.

Hypersplenism An overly active spleen, a normal function of which is to remove senescent platelets, red blood cells, and white blood cells from the circulation. If the organ is hyperactive, these cellular elements are removed while still normal.

Hypertension Abnormally high pressure; as used here, it refers to increased pressure in blood vessels.

Hypotension Abnormally low pressure; as used here, it refers to low blood pressure.

Icterus Jaundice.

Idiosyncratic An unpredictable hypersensitivity of an individual to a drug or food.

Ito cells Stellate cells.

Jaundice A yellowish color of tissue due to the deposit of bilirubin.

kg (kilogram) In the metric system, a unit of mass; 1 kilogram=2.2 pounds.

Lymphocyte An immune cell in blood and tissue. There are several types, but all are mononuclear, having a single round nucleus. Lymphocytes make up 20 to 30 percent of the white cells in human blood.

Macrophage A cell that takes in and destroys bacteria, particulate matter, or cell debris. There are multiple kinds of macrophages; some circulate in the bloodstream and others reside permanently in tissues.

Malaise A feeling of illness or a lack of energy; a symptom.

Mitochondria A structure in every living cell that produces the energy used by the cell.

ml or mL (milliliter) In the metric system, one thousandth of a liter, or approximately thirty drops.

Morbidity A measure of the changes in lifestyle made necessary by a disease; usually expressed as a rate of occurrence of such changes.

Mortality A measure of the rate of death associated with a disease or procedure.

Nausea A feeling that vomiting is about to occur.

Osmosis Movement of a solvent (e.g., water) through a semipermeable membrane (e.g., the membrane of a living cell) so that the concentrations of solutes (the material dissolved in the solvent) in the two solutions are equal.

Platelets Small cells circulating in blood that function to initiate clotting.

Polymorphonuclear Cells that have lobulated nuclei. These are the predominant form of white cells in blood, making up 65 to 75 percent of white cells in human blood.

Portal vein The major vein leading into the liver. All blood from the intestinal tract and spleen reaches the liver by this vein.

Prognosis An estimate or prediction of the outcome of a patient with an illness.

Prothrombin A protein necessary for blood to clot.

Sepsis Bacteria or their toxic products in blood. Sepsis represents a failure of the protective mechanisms of the body.

Sign An abnormality such as fever or an enlarged liver that is found during physical examination. Compare with "symptom."

Sinusoids (of liver) Tiny blood vessels making up the final division of the portal vein. Sinusoids, which do not have an epithelial lining, are surrounded by hepatic cells and are separated from them by a membrane. The space between the membrane and hepatic cells is called the space of Disse and is filled with serum that has a high concentration of albumin. Blood in sinusoids empties into hepatic veins.

Spider, hepatic A small cherry-red spot of blood vessels seen in those with liver disease. The "spider" represents a connection between an arteriole and a vein. These spots are found in patients with cirrhosis, although single ones can occasionally be seen in young people of child-bearing age without disease.

Splenomegaly Enlargement of the spleen.

Stellate cells Cells present in the liver which store vitamin A. When stimulated by cytokines, these cells begin secreting collagen to form fibrous tissue.

Stool Bowel movement; feces.

Symptom A complaint voiced by a patient.

Thrombophlebitis Inflammation of veins.

Umbilicus ("belly button") The point of attachment of the umbilical cord to the fetus. The umbilical artery and vein in the cord carry blood between the placenta and the baby.

Urobilinogen The breakdown product of bilirubin by bacteria in the colon. A portion is absorbed and excreted in urine.

Varices (esophageal) Dilated veins of the esophagus that become twisted and serpentine when forced to carry more blood than usual. (Varicose veins in the legs are an example of varices.)

Vena cava The largest vein in the body. It drains all blood from the lower extremities, passes underneath the liver, and empties into the right atrium of the heart.

Viremia Virus in the blood.

Warfarin A compound that binds vitamin K, preventing the formation of prothrombin and thus interfering with blood clotting. The form commonly used is Coumadin.

Xanthalasma An accumulation of cholesterol in the skin, forming a thick, yellowish plaque.

Index

Understanding Health and Sickness Series
Miriam Bloom, Ph.D., General Editor

Also in this series

Addiction • Alzheimer's Disease • Anemia • Asthma • Childhood Obesity • Chronic Pain • Colon Cancer • Crohn Disease and Ulcerative Colitis • Cystic Fibrosis • Dental Health • Depression • Herpes • Panic and Other Anxiety Disorders • Sickle Cell Disease